The Ultimate Lean Routine

The Ultimate Lean Routine

From the creator and director
of the Warner Bros. Fitness Center

Greg Isaacs

12-Week

Cross Training

& Fat Loss Program

THE SUMMIT PUBLISHING GROUP • ARLINGTON, TEXAS

THE SUMMIT PUBLISHING GROUP
One Arlington Centre
1112 East Copeland Road, Fifth Floor
Arlington, Texas 76011

Printed in the United States of America

96 97 98 99 00   011   5 4 3 2 1

Library of Congress Cataloging-in Publication Data

Isaacs, Greg, 1961-
    The ultimate lean routine: 12-week cross training and fat loss program / Greg Isaacs.
        p. cm.
    Includes index.
    ISBN 1-56530-203-6 (pbk. : alk. paper)
    1. Weight loss. 2. Reducing exercises. 3. Physical fitness.
I. Title
Rm222.2.I82
613.2'5--dc20   96-12350
                                                                                      CIP

A Note From The Publisher
The information herein is not intended to replace the services of trained health care professionals. You are advised to consult with your health care professional with regard to matters relating to your health and in particular, regarding matters which may require diagnosis or medical attention.

Cover and book design by David Sims
Cover Photography by Annette Buhl
Photography with text by Tracy Frankel

About The Author

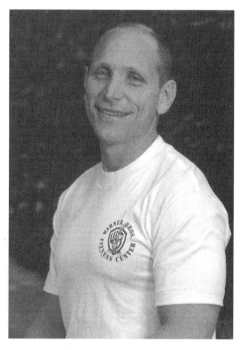

Greg Isaacs is the corporate fitness director for Warner Bros. Studios and a fitness consultant on high-profile projects such as the Time/Warner Resort in Acapulco and the Hard Rock Hotel in Las Vegas. Greg began his fitness career by introducing aerobics to South Africa, where he initiated the Instructor Certification Program. Building upon his studies in kinesiology and physical education, Greg maintains close contact with medical and scientific communities, and, together with his experience as a professional cyclist/triathlete, has developed his own principles of training and self-motivation. Greg works with many professional athletes and celebrities, including Bjorn Borg, Jimmy Connors, Melanie Griffith, Kurt Russell, Goldie Hawn, Don Johnson, Daniel Day-Lewis, John Lloyd, Kathy Smith, and Vendela. He believes that physical fitness is a great tool for developing self-confidence, managing stress, and achieving true inner health. Greg resides in Los Angeles with his wife, Diane, and two sons, Jackson and Wyatt.

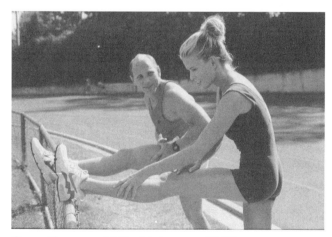

Greg with supermodel Vendela (see pages 73,74)

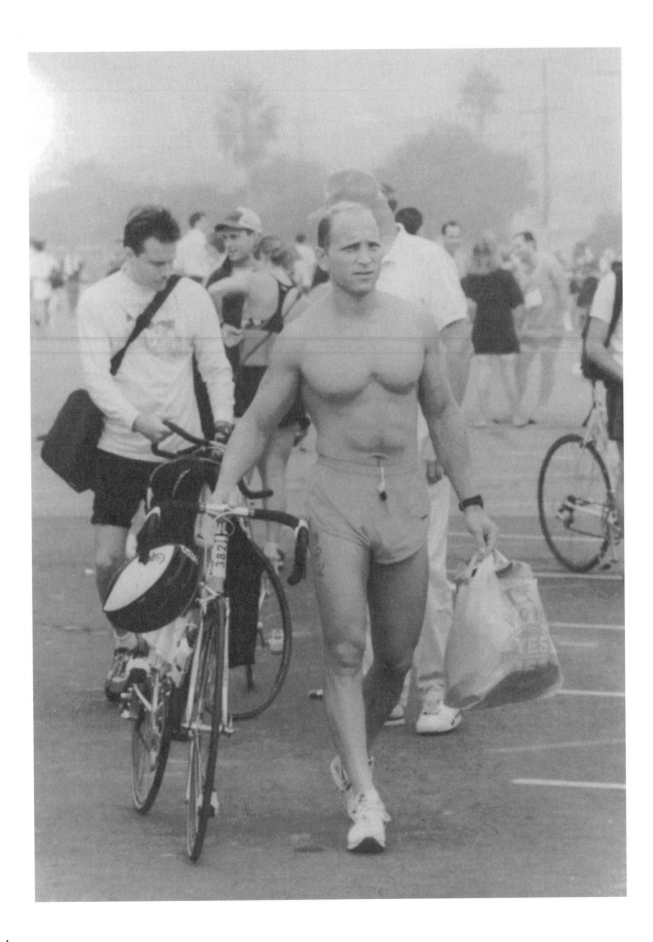

Table Of Contents

1 Goal Setting and the Systematic Approach to Fat Loss

There are few things in life more satisfying than setting and accomplishing a goal. When you think about it, much of our success in life is a result of our continuously setting and striving for new goals, both large and small. On the other hand, there are few things more disappointing than the failure to achieve a goal for which we have dreamed and worked hard. **Yet often what separate those of us who succeed from those who fail are little things like the possession of a bit more knowledge, a slightly better plan, or an ounce more of discipline.** The truth is that without the right formula or the appropriate action plan, even the simplest of goals can elude us. This is certainly true when it comes to fitness and fat loss. Although we all might intellectually recognize that total fitness is the result of nothing more than the right blend of diet, exercise, and rest, the truth is that figuring out the precise formula and then sticking with the plan can make the difference between success and failure. That's where this program can help you reach your goals. *The Ultimate Lean Routine* can guarantee success because it provides you both the formula and an easy-to-follow action plan.

▼
To ensure success, you have to start with a goal and the right formula.

Face it, despite an apparent wealth of information in all the media on training, fitness, weight loss, and nutrition, most of us actually know very little about exactly what's needed for us to achieve optimal fitness. We may have a tremendous amount of discipline and enthusiasm, but without the correct information, all the discipline in the world will do us no good. Moreover, an abundance of enthusiasm coupled with the wrong information can even get us into trouble. The vast majority of well-intentioned fitness enthusiasts have had no alternative but to haphazardly put together "personalized training programs" based only on random bits and pieces of information gathered from magazine articles, newspaper reports, television stories, and the advice of friends. **Until now, there has been no**

systematic scientific and easy approach to achieving a totally lean physique.

▼

After you know what exercises to do and how to eat properly, all you need to do is follow through.

The Ultimate Lean Routine was created to help you set and achieve your fat-loss and lean body-sculpting goals through the application of the same simple, scientifically proven cross-training principles that have been used successfully by world-class athletes for over a decade. This *Ultimate Lean Routine* manual explains cross-training and high-level fitness, guides you through a series of simple personal fitness evaluations, and allows you to monitor and motivate yourself using simple focused routines. **You'll learn exactly what workouts to do and how to eat every day.** The chapter on diet outlines a revolutionary approach to the tedious task of "counting calories and fat grams." It's called the IDEAL diet—IDEAL stands for "Individually Designed Eating Agenda and Lifestyle." On this program, you'll learn how to eat better every day instinctively to suit your own needs and not those of some nonexistent statistically average person. Finally, because our minds become more focused when objectives and goals are clearly spelled out, *The Ultimate Lean Routine* is designed as a practical twelve week project with a beginning, a middle, and an end. Once your twelve week personal project has been completed, you may choose to rest on your laurels, or you may choose to begin another twelve week cycle with even loftier goals. But either way, you'll probably never again allow yourself to train the way you did before reading *The Ultimate Lean Routine.*

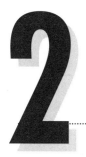 # Less Is More ...
(More or Less)

Although most fitness buffs believe that the more time they spend training, the better the results will be, the truth is that **the quality of both your workouts and your diet—not the quantity—determines the effectiveness of your program.** Despite the fact that disciplined individuals like bodybuilders or triathletes might think they need to spend upwards of thirty hours a week training every single muscle fiber in their bodies, the fact is this: **By selecting the correct workload, 90% of all possible training gains can be achieved in the first forty-five minutes of any workout.** You just have to know exactly what to do and how intensely to do it. Even more alarming is the fact that, in many cases, training more than ninety minutes in any one workout might not only impede your progress, but might actually set you back many days or even weeks—the very situation you want to avoid! Nothing can be more frustrating than putting in hours of training time and getting no results or—worse yet—getting negative results. *The Ultimate Lean Routine* was created to eliminate this frustration by preselecting only the most effective exercises and the ideal eating plan, and then outlining exactly what you do each day during the entire twelve week program. Each workout in *The Ultimate Lean Routine* was designed to produce maximum results and yet take less than an hour a day to complete. The emphasis is on quality—not quantity.

▼

Ninety percent of all training gains can be achieved in the first forty-five minutes of any workout if you know exactly what to do.

What to Expect from This Program

Before we proceed, it is important that you understand exactly what you can expect from *The Ultimate Lean Routine*. If, for some reason, you find that your own goals are other than those stated, you may want to reconsider beginning this program.

▼

Only cross-training and proper eating can create a truly fit person with low body fat, toned muscles, endurance, and flexibility.

The Ultimate Lean Routine makes the basic assumption that true fitness for both men and women combines **the best elements of low body fat, total body muscular strength, long and lean muscles, increased endurance, and better flexibility.** Training hard in just one discipline cannot result in all these things. Only cross-training and eating right can achieve these results. For example, bodybuilding in and of itself cannot result in total fitness. The effects of heavy weight training are too limiting, yielding only muscle mass without endurance. Similarly, running or cycling, while by themselves great endurance activities, fall short of producing total fitness. The optimum training program, *The Ultimate Lean Routine*, is a cross-training and ideal eating system intended to produce, after twelve weeks:

- Up to a 30% loss of body fat

- Up to a 50% increase in aerobic fitness

- Up to a 40% increase in muscle strength

- Longer, more sinewy muscle tone

- More energy

- More free time

The Basic Requirements

In order to get the most out of this program you'll need three things:

1. Membership in a gym or health club or access to a complete home gym. Without access to proper equipment, it is difficult to achieve the results listed earlier or to measure progress over time.

2. A reasonable starting level of fitness. This is not a program for absolute beginners. It's designed to take you to a new level of fitness. If you do not currently possess the fitness to routinely complete a one-hour aerobics class or ride a stationary bike for forty-five minutes without stopping, you should first check with your physician and, with his or her approval and guidance, spend several weeks building up an aerobic base before embarking on this or any other cross-training program.

3. The discipline to follow instructions and stick to the plan. *The Ultimate Lean Routine* will show you exactly what to do, but you still have to get out there and do it!

Step by Step

This manual will lead you step by step through the process of understanding fitness and gathering critical information about yourself. You will use this same information (weights, body fat percentages, training heart rates, etc.) to create your own unique training and IDEAL eating plan within the framework of *The Ultimate Lean Routine*. Your success with this program will depend on how closely you follow all the steps. Fortunately, each of the steps is easy to follow and to complete. Here are some general guidelines to help you get the most out of the program:

- **Read** this manual cover to cover.

- **Understand** all the concepts of fitness and fuel and how the body adapts to different training stimuli. Understanding helps your mind to stay focused on the program.

- **Record** all your essential personal starting data such as beginning body fat, lean body mass, personal caloric requirements, amounts of carbohydrates, fats, and protein, lactate threshold heart rate, lean training zone data, seat heights, Ten-rep Max, etc.

- **Set** realistic goals for the completion of the twelve week program based on your starting personal data.

- **Begin** your twelve week program with enthusiasm.

- **Log** and monitor your progress daily.

- **Follow through** with your commitment to yourself to do the best you can throughout the twelve weeks. A missed workout or an occasional off day will not impede you significantly as long as your relative progress continues over the twelve weeks.

- **Complete** the program, including the critical success evaluation sheets at the end of book.

- **Rest** completely or cut back for a week or two after completion of the program as a reward for a job well done.

Now let's get started.

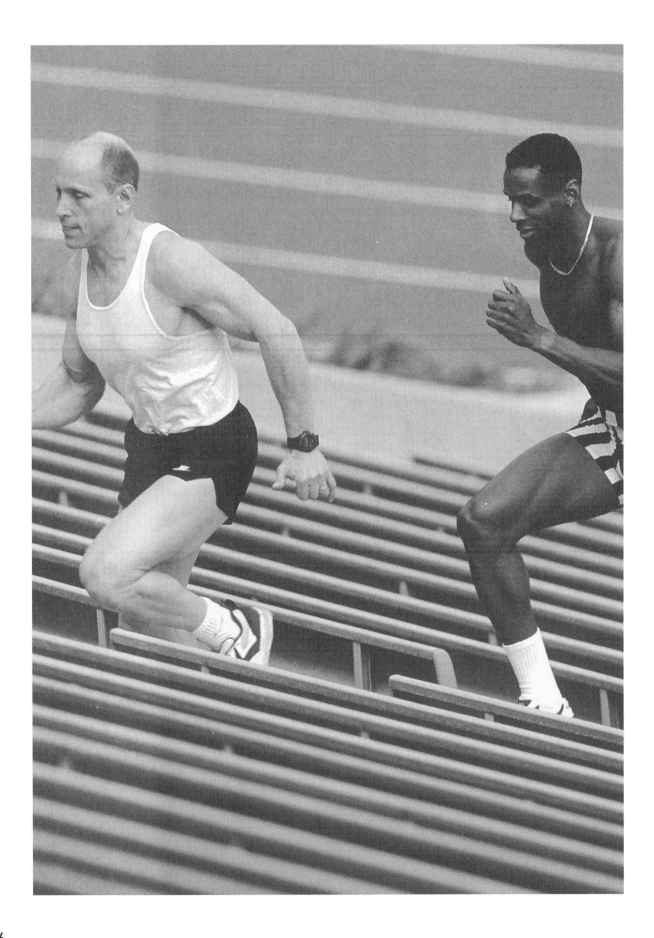

3 A Brief Look at How the Body Really Works

As stated previously, *The Ultimate Lean Routine* is based on important recent scientific research. What you will learn throughout this book is that some of this research may appear to conflict with some of the things you've read in popular magazines. In fact, you will begin to see that the fitness industry has occasionally even "misinterpreted" scientific results in order to sell fitness to an uninterested public. "Low-intensity workouts burn more fat" is an example of one such misinterpretation—they don't, in fact, but we'll talk more about that later. It will be necessary to explain and expose several common fitness "myths" in order to uncover the hard-core, results-oriented, bottom-line truth. But, as a result, you'll begin to understand what makes world-class athletes look as great and perform as well as they do. And you'll see how you can, too.

There's a Little Tarzan (or Jane) in Each of Us

The human body is a product of evolution. We each represent the result of millions of years of random genetic mutations and specific individual adaptations to a hostile environment. Our ability to run long distances, to sprint, to lift heavy weights, and to store and burn fats is the result of our remote ancestors having been "fit" enough to survive the challenges of this hostile environment and pass their genes along to us. Thanks (or no thanks) to modern technology, many of those essential survival adaptations serve little or no purpose today. Unlike our ancestors, we are no longer forced to live off our stored fat as we migrate hundreds of miles to new sources of food. Instead, when the refrigerator is empty, we just drive on down to the corner supermarket and load up. Unlike our ancestors, we haven't been forced to sprint to safety several times a day— unless, maybe, when crossing a New York City street. You can see the point: Our

▼

Evolution has allowed us to become fat today, but evolution can also allow us to become extremely fit tomorrow.

basic survival is pretty well assured. However, as a result of all this technology, our species has become very soft. In many respects we have devolved from our primal ancestors' high level of fitness.

▼

The challenge of training is to identify the exact stress necessary to cause a desired adaptation. This general adaptation principle is the main reason training works.

Fortunately, all of us share the same basic biochemical mechanisms that our ancestors used to survive their hostile environment. These same biological mechanisms still allow certain **adaptations** to take place over time that can make us faster, stronger, and leaner. All of the necessary information is contained in the DNA of each of our cells—the same DNA that has been passed down for millions of years. These DNA blueprints are immediately available to guide or create a specific adaptation whenever we choose the appropriate stimulus. Our challenge is to identify the kind of **adaptation** we want to produce (more speed, less body fat, longer and stronger muscles, etc.) and then select an appropriate **stress** (or stimulus) that will cause the body to generate the desired adaptation. Scientists often refer to this as the "general adaptation principle." Stated another way, if we take any living organism, cell system, or even an enzyme or hormonal system, and we apply a specific stress, and then we allow the cell or organism time to recover, it will adapt to that stress—that is, it will become better able to handle the stress the next time the stress is present.

STRESS + REST = POSITIVE ADAPTATION

For instance, most of us already know that in order to stimulate general muscle growth, we must place a significant stress on muscle cells by adding progressive resistance. Lifting weights is a common application of this simple principle. Likewise, in order to be able to run a marathon, we must stress certain leg muscle fibers and energy systems by progressively increasing both the distance and speed of our runs. Yet marathon training is very different from the training a sprinter would choose, even though both involve strengthening the muscles of the legs. In each case, the body makes very specific biological changes (adaptations) due to different chemical signals released from the muscles as a result of each particular stress.

Because running sprints produces chemical signals that are quite different from those produced by running long distances, it's no wonder that a wide receiver looks entirely different from a marathoner. With the human body, as with architectural design, "form follows function." The shape our body takes will be a direct result of the type of specific adaptation or function we've chosen. For this reason, a distance runner generally has a smaller upper body because runners have no functional requirement for big chests and arms. But distance runners do have long, powerful legs for obvious reasons. Likewise, the "racquet" arm of a tennis player is sometimes twice as big around as the opposite, less-used arm; a powerlifter may be big and strong but often has as much as 30 or 40 percent body fat because there's no functional reason for him (or her) not to be fat.

You might then think that just picking out the right type of stimulus and training like a fiend for twelve weeks would result in form following function all the way to your ultimate goal. There's a hitch, though. **You need to select a specific stimulus that is just enough to cause a desired adaptation but not so great that it causes damage.** The German philosopher Friedrich Nietzsche put it in the most blunt of terms when he said, "That which does not kill me makes me stronger." If the stress or stimulus is too frequent or too intense, not only does the organism (or cell or enzyme system) not adapt, it also may become injured or damaged.

One of the clearest illustrations of the general adaptation principle at work is the stress/adaptation effect of sunlight on skin. We all know that a brief exposure to sunlight causes no adaptation, because the stress is not enough to generate a response; a slightly longer exposure (an appropriate stress), followed by rest, results in the mobilization of melanin pigments to the skin's surface (also known as a tan) which has the effect of helping to block some of the light's penetration at a later time. In effect, the skin becomes better able to handle the stress the next time it comes around. It adapts to the stress. However, if we bombard unadapted fair skin with a prolonged exposure to the sun's rays, that skin becomes damaged, and we have what we call a "sunburn." In this case, the stress is just too great. When that happens, we set our intended adaptation back several days or weeks. Consequently, we must avoid any further exposure to sunlight in order to allow the damaged tissue to heal. Only then, after the skin has healed, can we begin the adaptive process all over again.

▼

If a training stress is not intense enough, no adaptation occurs and the body undergoes no change in form.

This same principle applies to fitness training: If a training stress is not enough to stimulate the body to adapt, nothing happens. We often encounter this in the gym when we see people doing the same workout we've seen them do every day for months with no results. They might be riding the bike at the same level for the same amount of time or lifting the same weights they've lifted for years. In effect, these people's bodies have already adapted to that particular amount of stress. The same stress (the same old workout) is no longer enough to stimulate further adaptation. It's no wonder these people get frustrated. They're obviously putting the time in, but unless they do something to give the body a reason to adapt, unless they boost the intensity, they're doomed to see no new progress.

▼

If a training stress is too great, severe damage can result.

On the other hand, if the stress we select is too great or if the rest period not long enough, severe damage can be done, from which it might take weeks to recover. For example, having an untrained person attempt to run six or seven miles in the first workout would have this effect, as would something as supposedly harmless as simply training a little too long or a little too hard every day for a few weeks. This latter scenario, familiar to many triathletes and other gung-ho workout fanatics, is known as "chronic overtraining." **Selecting the proper types and amounts of stress and rest is the essence of all fitness training and is the most important principle behind** *The Ultimate Lean Routine.*

One other important element of the general adaptation principle has to do with food. As we will see shortly, your IDEAL diet—the fuel you choose—is critical to both the rest and the stress elements of our equation. Adequate fuel supplies ensure that when we do apply stress to the muscles, there are sufficient energy reserves to generate the desired response and that, later, when we rest, the muscles have all the necessary "building materials" to create the desired adaptation. Without proper fuel, even the best exercise action plan is doomed to failure.

As a result, our revised training equation should look like this:

Stress (exercise) + rest (recovery time and IDEAL diet) =
positive adaptation (strength and fat loss)

Ipso Fatso—Bad News and Good News

First the bad news: As a survival-oriented organism, the human body has always had the **conservation of energy** as its primary order of business. Under normal circumstances, our bodies will automatically take every opportunity possible to store energy rather than expend it. This is because the most primitive part of our brain is "hard-wired" to instruct us both biochemically and behaviorally to avoid any expenditures of energy that are not absolutely necessary for survival. As a result of this survival adaptation, we have an alarmingly efficient ability to store any excess calories we eat as body fat, rather than to burn them off immediately after they are consumed. This automatic tendency to conserve energy explains why most of the human population prefers to sit around the house doing nothing all day. It also explains why our doing the same workout routine day in and day out will yield little or no additional result; energy must be spent for the body to create any adaptation. After an adaptation to a particular amount of work has been made, the body can "coast" at that new level and **conserve** its energy. Therefore, we have to continuously "trick" the body into making new adaptations.

And now the good news: Fortunately for this program, we all carry with us the necessary DNA blueprints to teach our bodies how to burn fat with reckless abandon, provided we give our bodies the appropriate fat-burning stresses. We also have a neocortex in our brain that allows us to use our willpower to bypass or override that hard-wired couch potato in us and to suppress those survival thoughts that might cause us to want to walk instead of run or to take a nap instead of work out.

▼

Fortunately, with a little will-power and the right type of training we can learn to burn off most of our fat.

Every Body Is Different

Obviously men and women have several slight anatomical differences that will lead to slightly different degrees of adaptation throughout *The Ultimate Lean Routine*. Generally, men have a higher metabolism than women. This means that over the course of a day men burn more calories workload for workload and can consume more calories to maintain a stable body fat and lean body mass. A greater abundance of male "androgenic" hormones will also cause men to build a little more muscle and become a little stronger. On the other hand, women tend to adapt to burning body fat a little better than men, although they do so at a lower rate of fuel use. Also, women have a basic requirement for more body fat than men. Survival adaptations over the eons have resulted in women's maintaining an extra supply of adipose tissue over the hips and around the breasts. But the fact remains that men and women still burn fuel and respond to both aerobic and anaerobic exercise the same way.

The net effect of this difference is that we cannot compare "hardbody" men to "hardbody" women using a similar body fat standard. Whereas 10% body fat would be considered excellent for a twenty-five-year-old man, that same 10% would be a dangerously low level for a woman.

Factoring in her gender-specific fat requirements, an excellent standard for a woman the same age is probably closer to 17% or 18%. Although body fat percentages under those levels might qualify you as "ripped" at the gym, the fact is that very low fat levels are considered "less than healthy" and can become dangerous at under 5% or 6% for men and 9% or 10% for women.

It is also true that there are certain family history or genetic differences among us that can limit the speed or extent to which we respond to these fitness stresses or stimuli. Some women and men will just drop fat far more rapidly than others; some will build muscle quicker. But the bottom line is that whatever the degree of change in one person vs. another, the basic principles—and the biological mechanisms by which they work—still apply to everyone across the board.

Exercise physiologists speak of the three basic body "types" that are used to describe genetic differences among individuals. These body types are ectomorphs, mesomorphs, and endomorphs. As a rule, endomorphs tend to have thicker bones and to deposit more body fat (and have more trouble keeping it off). Mesomorphs are apt to be more muscular and to have less body fat. Ectomorphs tend to be the skinniest among us, with less muscle and less fat.

In reality, however, no one is 100% ectomorph, mesomorph, or endomorph. We are all various blends of these characteristics because over generations, the genetic pool is continually mixed. Nevertheless, someone who tends more toward the endomorphic side needs to understand that he or she may never be able to reach 8% or 12% body fat and still maintain good health. For those men who are predominantly endomorphic, a body fat level of 15% will look and feel great, as will 24% on an endomorphic woman. Similarly, someone with mostly ectomorphic qualities may never achieve those twenty-one-inch biceps he or she is seeking. Nevertheless, armed with this knowledge, and knowing a little about our parents and grandparents, we can each better assess our individual potential and arrive at goals that are both realistic and achievable.

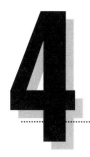

Energy Systems: Food = Fuel

The body uses fuel to accomplish its work in much the same way that an engine uses fuel to run. We just happen to derive all of our fuel from the foods we eat. The conversion of these food units to fuel units takes place in the stomach, liver, and small intestine through a process known as digestion. The end products of this breakdown of food are three basic types of fuel—fat, protein, and carbohydrate—each of which provides a different "octane" and burns at a distinctly different rate. Yet each is absolutely essential to our performance and our ability to get rid of stored fat.

In order to do any exercise, whether it's a quick sprint, a long swim, a high jump, a heavy lift, or just getting out of the chair to go to the refrigerator for a beer, a chain reaction of complex fuel-driven events must take place. First, the brain must send a set of signals to the appropriate muscles instructing them to contract. It uses fuel (in this case, glucose) to help generate the transmission of those signals. When the signals arrive from the brain, tiny **myofilaments,** the smallest units of muscle, start to contract. Millions of these tiny myofilaments are involved in the contraction of each muscle fiber and thousands of muscle fiber contractions in each complete large muscle movement or repetition of an exercise. The chemical that directly causes all this contraction is adenosine triphosphate or "ATP." Each time a muscle fiber is called upon by the brain to contract, several molecules of ATP **must** be present in order to fuel the contraction of each single myofilament. Without ATP, no muscle movement could take place. This "universal" fuel could make for a very simple system if it were not for one big drawback: Our muscles never contain more than a very small amount of ATP. In fact, at any given time we each have only enough ATP to run all out for a little more than ten seconds. Imagine if we had to rely just on our limited ATP for all our living requirements; we would need to

▼

Without the three essential food "fuels"—fat, carbohydrate, and protein— burning stored fat is almost impossible.

get used to the idea of collapsing in a heap every time our ATP was used up, until enough ATP could somehow be remanufactured to fuel another ten seconds of activity. Some lifestyle! Fortunately, we have adapted to get around this dilemma by continuously "recycling" the small amount of ATP we do have, using the three better known fuels that are present in large amounts in the foods we eat. We know these fuels as **fat, carbohydrate, and protein.** Of course, these also happen to be the very same fuels we obsess over for their various caloric contents!

Each of these three fuels allows us to recycle ATP at different rates and with different degrees of "efficiency," depending on how intensely we are working. It follows that if we know a little about how each fuel functions, we can better determine just how much of each fuel we need to consume daily and which exercises will best work with these fuels to cause the loss of body fat and the growth of muscle tissue.

Carbohydrates
High octane, but low "miles per gallon," limited storage capacity

When muscles run out of stored carbohydrate, they stop working.

Carbohydrates (also known as "carbs") have gotten a bad rap over the years, but for many of the wrong reasons. The prevalent misconception was that carbohydrates were bad because they immediately became stored fat. Although it is true that carbohydrates can be converted to fat when eaten in excess or when not burned off (as happens all too easily with sedentary people), the truth is that carbohydrates are the most important source of fuel for fit people. Our muscles perform very efficiently burning carbohydrates (and, as a result, recycling ATP) at all levels of activity from very low level aerobic workouts to the most intense anaerobic activities. Carbohydrate is so critical to muscular work that **when muscles run out of their stored form of carbohydrate, muscular work ceases completely. In fact, this is what happens when runners "hit the wall."** Despite the fact that a runner hitting the wall still might have lots of stored fat fuel remaining, carbohydrates **must** be present in order for those fats to be metabolized. This is why exercise physiologists say that "fat burns in a carbohydrate flame."

The carbohydrates in the food we eat are broken down by the stomach and liver and are eventually converted to **glucose.** Some becomes available for immediate use by muscles and the brain (the other major glucose consumer). **Excess carbohydrate can be stored as glycogen in the muscles**

and the liver for later use. However, after these glycogen storage areas are full, most remaining carbohydrate gets converted to fat. Because our bodies can store only very limited amounts of glycogen and because we tap into this glycogen supply so often during the day, **regular carbohydrate consumption is vital to athletic performance**. It is ironic that carbohydrate represents such an ideal fuel because even a well-trained endurance athlete can store only enough carbohydrate (in the form of glycogen) in the muscles and liver to run for a maximum of two hours. After that, or much sooner in untrained individuals, glycogen depletion causes a dramatic plunge in performance—known as "the wall"—which can cause the body to "cannibalize" itself for survival if the effort is continued. Total carbohydrate storage capacity in the liver and muscles ranges from just 200 to 500 grams (about 800 to 2,000 calories' worth) of glycogen, a fact we will use later to help plan our daily carbohydrate intake.

Under ideal conditions, active individuals would eat small amounts of carbohydrate throughout the day, "grazing" just enough to provide a constant supply of this muscle fuel to give us a steady level of energy without tapping into our glycogen reserves, altering our blood glucose levels, or causing us to store any excess carbohydrate as fat. In reality, because most of us eat once only every several hours, what often happens is that we "gorge" ourselves on carbohydrates, especially simple sugars. This can start a cascade of undesirable events that leads to low energy and more stored fat (*see Fig. 1*)! First, as the glucose levels in the blood rise immediately after the meal, we feel "wired," almost overly energized, for a brief period of time. With this rise in glucose, a chemical signal is sent to the pancreas to secrete insulin, a hormone whose function is to be certain we don't waste any of this precious fuel (survival and fuel conservation, remember?). Insulin works to take much of the excess glucose out of the bloodstream and put it into the cells, where it can be stored as glycogen **and stored as fat**—not exactly our goal in *The Ultimate Lean Routine*. Furthermore, this over reaction on the part of the pancreas secreting insulin often takes so much glucose out of the bloodstream that our blood glucose soon plummets below optimal and we begin to feel tired, weak, and lightheaded. Remember that the brain functions only on glucose, and here we have suddenly removed a great deal of this "brain fuel" from the bloodstream. Because the brain also controls our willingness to work out, any motivation to train is now gone. The final insult is that, with this new drop in blood glucose, more chemical sensors actually instruct the brain to make

▼

Eating complex carbohydrates and "grazing" are two keys to maintaining energy and burning fat.

us hungry again so that we eat enough to raise the blood glucose level (survival again). These wide swings in blood glucose (also known as blood sugar) can put us on a moody high-low roller coaster, sapping us of energy while adding unnecessary fat storage. This is a lifestyle and eating style to which far too many Americans fall victim. Obviously then, how and when we eat carbohydrates, and the types of carbohydrates we eat, can play a crucial role in our energy levels, our fat storage, and our fat burning!

One of the keys to maintaining a steady flow of carbohydrate is to consume most of your carbs in the form of complex carbohydrates—as opposed to simple carbohydrates (or simple sugars). Complex carbohydrates are foods that contain long chains of sugars that take a while to break down in the stomach and are released slowly and steadily into the bloodstream to supply a more uniform level of blood glucose well after they are consumed. This reduces the amount of insulin released by the pancreas, which in turn reduces the amount of glucose that gets converted into fat and stored in the fat cells. On the other hand, simple sugars—like those found in many processed foods, breakfast cereals, desserts, and other sweets—break down very rapidly. Although this process can be favorable under certain limited circumstances (like when you are fifty miles into a bike ride or two hours into a run and your glycogen reserves are completely depleted), more often the result of our eating simple sugars is that we just store as fat what we don't immediately burn off. Obviously, if we want to avoid a fat-storing situation we should steer clear of simple sugars and seek out complex carbohydrates whenever possible.

Complex carbohydrates are found in most starches, grains, pastas, breads, and in the fibrous parts of many vegetables. A diet high in grains and vegetables would provide for plenty of complex carbohydrates.

The other key is to spread your carbohydrate consumption out over the day, avoiding single large carbohydrate meals in favor of smaller and more frequent meals or snacks. We'll get into exactly how to plan this shortly.

Protein
Almost no octane, very low "miles per gallon"; primarily for growth, maintenance, and repair; for use as fuel only in cases of emergency

The main function of protein is to supply amino acids for a variety of bodily functions, the most noteworthy of which is for the formation of muscle tissue, also known as lean body mass. Protein is responsible for

Fig. 1

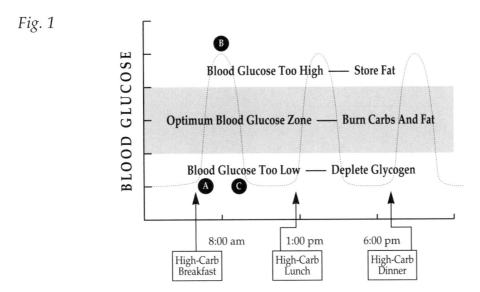

WRONG!

1. The typical American diet seems to consist of three big meals a day. If these meals contain too much carbohydrate, especially simple sugars, the effect can be a devastating emotional and energy roller coaster. Almost immediately after a high-carbohydrate meal (A) the blood glucose level rises above the optimum zone and we feel wired and energetic—but only briefly. When blood glucose hits a certain point, (B) the pancreas dumps insulin into the bloodstream. This insulin causes the rapid removal of glucose from the blood. Some of the removed glucose is stored as glycogen, some is stored as fat, but the drastic drop in blood glucose causes us to feel weak, light-headed, tired—and hungry again. (C) Another high carbohydrate meal starts the process all over again.

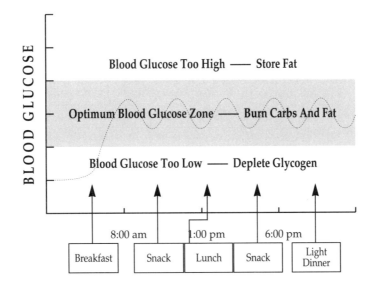

RIGHT!

2. By eating a better mix of protein, carbohydrate, and fat at each meal, by sticking with complex carbs instead of simple sugars, and by "grazing" with smaller main meals and healthy snacks, it is possible to keep blood glucose within an optimum zone all day. The result: a steady supply of energy and far less stored fat.

maintaining and repairing our muscular and skeletal structure, and is not a readily available fuel to be burned for energy. Recently, there has been a re-examination of the importance of protein in our diets, and the recommended daily allowance of protein has been debated among health experts. Some argue that our needs for protein have greatly diminished through evolution due to modern conveniences, while others believe that we have the genetic predisposition from early man that requires high levels of protein. Regardless of the conflicting philosophies, protein is an essential food in achieving a lean body.

The U.S. Recommended Daily Allowance is .8 grams of protein per kg of body weight per day. However, research has shown that athletes in particular may require twice the RDA, and those that actively exercise, may need more as well. Inadequate protein in your diet can lead to muscle breakdown and loss, a dietary imbalance, and reduced exercise performance. It may be the missing element that keeps many of us from achieving greater muscle definition and lower body fat percentages. Without replenishing the muscles worked with protein, the muscle tissue is broken down by the mechanical and metabolic stresses of exercises. Protein is the key dietary portion of the "rest" in our equation of "positive adaptation". It restores and builds the muscle mass while increasing results and enhancing your performance.

Under normal resting conditions, we derive only 1% to 2% of our total fuel (ATP recycling) requirements from protein metabolism. Protein's contribution to energy becomes significant only under circumstances that the body recognizes (yet again) as "survival situations." One such example occurs when we exercise vigorously for more than an hour or two without taking in any fuel during the exercise. In this case, as glycogen stores become depleted from muscle and the liver, the body actually begins to break down its own muscle tissue to supply more glucose to the remaining working muscles. Although this "self-cannibalization" might make some sense from a purely survival point of view, it is hardly productive for an athlete or other fitness buff trying to build muscle for the future! The best way to avoid this situation is to never reach a glycogen-depleted state, either by making sure you consume adequate carbs and limiting your intense exercise routines to less than two hours, or by continuously taking in carbohydrate fuel during longer bouts of exercise.

The other example of protein's use as emergency fuel occurs during starvation, deprivation, or very low-calorie diets. In these cases, the body

▼

Normal diets don't work because they cause the body to conserve fat and burn muscle.

18

recognizes the lack of adequate food as a survival emergency and, in an effort to conserve energy, lowers the body's metabolism and again cannibalizes muscle tissue to provide more glucose for the brain. What's even more alarming, under this situation the body actually attempts to conserve fat as well! It's important to understand that under extreme starvation conditions, the body regards active muscle tissue (the largest consumer of energy in the body) as a liability. It naturally attempts to dispose of this liability. Unfortunately, this fact is precisely why diet programs alone don't work. The dieter succeeds only in losing water and all-important lean muscle, while at the same time lowering his or her metabolism. The results are: less energy to exercise, less muscle tissue to actually do any exercise, and a tendency to store more fat after the caloric restrictions are lifted because less muscle tissue now means it takes fewer calories to maintain "normal" weight.

The key consideration is this: On a daily basis we need to know how much energy in the form of carbohydrates and fats we will need to provide fuel for our muscles. Then, when figuring out our daily protein requirements, we need to concern ourselves with our body's requirement for growth and maintenance. Oftentimes, it is difficult to ingest extra protein in your diet, therefore I recommend the use of a protein powder to achieve your protein requirements. We'll discuss how to figure your personal needs in the next chapter.

Fats
Low octane, high "miles per gallon" but only at slow speeds, unlimited storage capacity

Fats have become the taboo fuel of the 90s. Depending on whom you debate, fats are responsible for all the ills of society from cancer to heart disease. To a certain extent, this is true. An excess consumption of fat is considered one of the worst nutritional mistakes we can make. Nevertheless, fats also serve a purpose as one of the most important fuels athletes have at their disposal.

▼

At rest, a fit person gets 75%-90% of all energy from burning stored fat.

Fat is a major fuel source for basic metabolic maintenance. Some studies have shown that, at rest, a fit individual derives 75% to 90% of all energy requirements from the slow burning of fats. This alone tends to validate the observation that someone with a so-called "high metabolism" will generally be blessed with low body fat. He or she simply burns fat off all day. Fat also provides a layer of thermal insulation under the skin.

Anthropologists will tell us that this served an important survival purpose in the days before clothing was invented. Obviously, carrying our own thermal insulation is not a survival necessity any longer! Finally, some amount of dietary fat is essential for the production of certain hormones and other regulatory chemicals.

Fats are best known to athletes as aerobic fuel. As a result, athletes are constantly training their bodies to burn fats aerobically as a way of reducing their dependency on their limited glycogen reserves (remember that after you're out of glycogen, the race is over). Given the right conditions (as in: lots of oxygen present and very low levels of continuous activity) fat can account for a huge amount of ATP recycling. In fact, under ideal conditions, one molecule of fat will yield 441 molecules of ATP. By contrast, one molecule of carbohydrate burned aerobically will yield just thirty-six molecules of ATP, and the same carbohydrate molecule burned anaerobically will yield only two molecules of ATP! Using this analysis, you can see that fat is an extremely efficient fuel. That's great if you are trying to survive off the land or are competing in a thousand-mile walking race, but not so great if you are trying to diminish your fat reserves on one hour a day of training!

▼

Intensity is the key to training. The more calories you burn in a given period of time, the more fat you'll lose.

From a performance point of view, the higher the intensity of activity, the less **relative** contribution fat can make to the ATP energy recycling effort. That's because at higher intensities there's not nearly enough oxygen available to allow fat to burn aerobically and still provide all energy needs. Consider this comparison: Whereas someone walking briskly might derive 60% of all calories from the burning of fats, and most of the balance of energy from carbohydrates, someone running fairly hard might get only 30% of total calories from fats and the other 70% from carbs. Sounds like you burn more fats going slower, right? Wrong. This is a fact that the fitness industry has used erroneously to preach that low levels of aerobic activity are the best way to burn fats. In reality, **the most important factor in losing fat is the total amount of calories burned during the exercise.** The more calories you burn in a given amount of time—whether from carbs, fat, or even protein—the more fat you will eventually lose. Intensity is the key. This is because long after you finish exercising more intensely, the body continues to burn fat at a much higher rate than it normally would at rest. Let's look at our example (*Fig. 2*): Someone walking at an easy pace of 300 calories per hour might "burn" 180 calories' worth of fat during the walk (60% of 300). In contrast, someone running at a moderately intense rate might derive

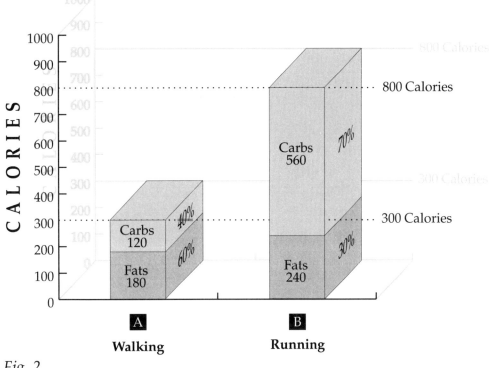

Fig. 2

A *walks at 3 MPH for sixty minutes. While 60% of all calories being burned is from fat, the total calories burned in the hour is only 300.*

B *runs at 7 MPH for sixty minutes. Even though "relatively" less fat percentage is being burned, the total amount of fat burned is higher and the total calories burned is more than twice as high for the same amount of time spent exercising. Furthermore, B will burn more fat during the next few hours of rest as his/her body replaces lost glycogen.*

only 30% of the total calories from burning fat, but he or she is burning 800 calories per hour, so the person will still burn 240 calories of fat during the hour. In addition, the same person will burn another 560 calories' worth of carbohydrate during the run. And furthermore—and this is the key to higher intensity workouts—that person will **continue to burn fats at a higher rate for several hours after the run is over** as the body uses some of its stored fat to help replace the lost glycogen! If low-intensity workouts were the only way to burn fat, wouldn't it make sense that sprinters (who never do low-intensity workouts) would be fat? Obviously, they're not. Sprinters have some of the lowest body fat in the exercising population. **Recent studies confirm that cross-training moderately to intensely not only can cause you to burn more calories during a workout, but also can elevate your resting metabolic rate by as much as 11%.** To put it another way, the proper cross-training plan can cause you to burn 11% more fat while you're just sitting around the house doing nothing!

▼

Moderately intense exercise "teaches" the body to take fat out of adipose tissue and move it to muscle tissue, where it can be more easily burned during the next workout.

One other "benefit" of fat as a fuel, quite unfortunately, is our ability to store large amounts of it in the form of "adipose tissue" on our waist, under our arms, and on our hips, butts, and thighs. In fact, even a very fit 160-pound man with only 7% body fat (considered very low by anyone's standards) still has enough stored fat to theoretically walk three hundred miles without refueling. We say "theoretically" because the biggest drawback to having this stored fat is our inefficiency at taking our fat out of storage and getting it quickly to the muscles where it can be burned. The good news, according to recent laboratory research, is that after a few weeks of moderately intense exercise (such as we will be doing in this program), the body "learns" to take some fat out of adipose storage while we rest and deposit it directly in the muscles, where it can be more easily burned during the next session of exercise. Obviously, this fat transfer from adipose tissue to storage in the muscles works to our advantage if we are seeking to squander our stored fat!

One final limitation to fat as fuel, which we discussed earlier, is the fact that fat can burn only in the presence of oxygen and only when carbohydrate is also being burned. Therefore, a key point to remember is: **If you want to burn fat efficiently, always make sure your carbohydrate levels are adequate.** We will use this fact later when we design our eating "schedule."

▼

We all carry enough stored fat that we shouldn't have to eat much additional fat to maintain energy or health.

In practical terms, because we all have such an excellent ability to store fat, and because excess carbohydrate (and even excess protein) can be converted to fat, **we really don't need to consume a lot of fat to sustain energy levels.** In fact, this is what virtually all health-related organizations and governmental agencies agree on: We generally eat far too much fat and should take whatever steps necessary to cut back on fat consumption. If you can limit your intake of fat to 20% or less of your total calories, you'll get the best results from this program.

So, exactly how much of this stored fuel are you carrying around and how much can you afford to lose? Read on.

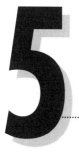

Getting a Handle on Your Stored Fat

One of the problems with stored fat is that it is not metabolically active. That is, no matter how much fat you have on your body, it does not burn calories. Fat is just stored fuel. **Only metabolically active tissue like your muscles, brain, and other organs can actually burn calories throughout the day. This metabolically active tissue is called "lean body mass" (LBM).** To simplify, lean body mass consists of all of you that is not fat. The formula for determining lean body mass is simple, provided you know your weight and the percentage of you that is fat:

Body weight (pounds) – fat mass (pounds) = lean body mass (pounds)

When you begin to think in terms of lean body mass vs. fat, you will begin to see why standard height and weight charts are not necessarily a good way to determine whether you are "fit" or at the appropriate weight. For example, consider two men, both 5'10", both weighing 180 pounds, both "outside" the normal healthy standards on a chart. However, a closer look reveals that one of these men is quite muscular, has only 10% body fat, and is extremely fit and healthy. The other has 30% body fat and is truly unfit and unhealthy. Their height and weight may be the same, but without our knowing their body fat percentages, we cannot predict their fitness levels or general health from a standard height and weight chart.

In another example, a 5'8" well-muscled, 135-pound woman with 16% body fat may be as fit and healthy and look as great as a slightly leaner, "svelte" 5'8" 125-pound woman with the same 16% body fat, even though the one weighs ten pounds more than the other. Same height, same body fat, same degree of fitness. The difference is LBM (lean body mass)—approximately six extra pounds of muscle and 2.4 extra pounds of bone on the heavier, more "muscled woman." (*The 135-pound woman, at 16% body fat, is 84% lean body mass or 113.4 pounds; the 125-pound woman has the same 84% lean body mass of her 125-pound total weight or 105 pounds. The difference is 8.4 pounds.*) All of this can be explained through either genetic differences or through different training regimens.

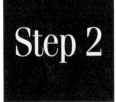

Step 1

Weigh yourself.

Weighing Yourself

Knowing your total body weight is essential in order to determine your lean body mass, how much actual fat you have, and how much you can afford to lose. So the first step is to weigh yourself. Keep in mind that, whenever you weigh yourself throughout this program, you should do so on the same scale, with little or no clothing, and at the same time of day, because this will give you the most accurate picture of your relative progress.

Weight in pounds = _____

Step 2

Determine your body fat percentage.

Measuring Starting Body Fat

In order to judge the effectiveness of any fat-loss program, it's crucial that you accurately measure your starting body fat—not just your weight—and monitor the progressive loss of fat throughout the program. The problem is that this process is usually quite expensive, time-consuming, and can even be a little humiliating if you do it at a gym or physician's office. As a result, many people never get a clue as to their true body fat. Or if they do, it's information they might get only once every few years. To fill this void, some versions of this program include one of the most simple, yet accurate, body fat-measuring devices available. Because the majority of fat on the body is stored directly under the skin, using this skinfold measurement device can be as accurate and reliable as more expensive electronic or water tank (hydrostatic weighing) methods. The Easy-Measure calipers enable you to quickly, easily, and privately measure body fat as often as you want. If your program did not include these calipers, you may order some directly or through one of the many fitness magazines and catalogs that carry body fat calipers. Or you can have your physician, club, or gym test your body fat for you.

If you do have calipers, do your measuring standing up and wearing loose (or no) clothing. Start by making sure the slide element is all the way over to the right. Then simply find your right iliac crest (top of right hipbone) and firmly pinch the skin just an inch above it between your left thumb and forefinger *(Photo 1)*.

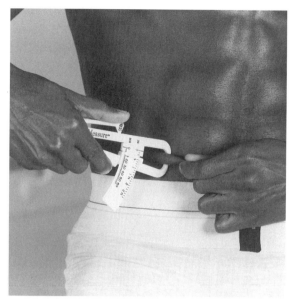

Photo 1

Place the jaws of the calipers over the skinfold while continuing to hold the skinfold with your left hand. Now press with the thumb where it's indicated on the Easy-Measure until you feel a slight click. The slide member will automatically stop at the correct measurement. After reading your measurement, return the slide member to the far right starting position. Repeat this two more times and use the average as your measurement. Refer to the body fat interpretation chart on page 176 to determine your exact body fat percentage. Now that you know your body fat percentage, you will record it as a starting point in the beginning of your logbook and then again once every two weeks during the twelve week program.

If you do not have skin calipers, I have included a chart to calculate your body fat percentage.

Men
1. Measure your weight to the nearest pound.
2. Measure your waist circumference at the level of your navel, for your Lower Abdominal Girth
3. Align a straight-edged ruler with your WEIGHT and LOWER ABDOMINAL GIRTH measurements on the corresponding columns.
4. Read your body fat percentage at the point the ruler crosses the column.

Women
1. Measure your height to the nearest .25 inches.
2. Measure circumference of your hips with a tape measure at the level of your hip bones, for your girth.
3. Align a straight-edged ruler with your height and hip girth measurements on the corresponding columns.

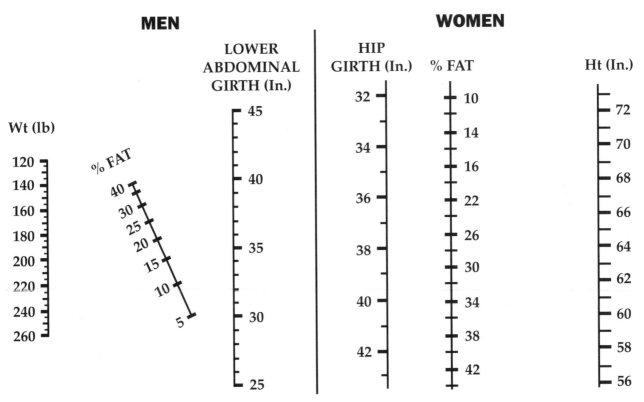

MEN   **WOMEN**

4. Read your body fat percentage at the point the ruler crosses the column.

Body fat = _____ %

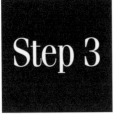

Step 3

Calculate how much your stored body fat weighs.

Calculating Body Fat in Pounds

Next, to get an idea of just how much fat you are carrying around and how much you can realistically lose, it will be necessary to plug the numbers into your equation for "total body fat in pounds." Determine the amount of fat you are carrying by multiplying:

Current weight _____(pounds) x _____% body fat *(from preceding measurement)*
= _____ pounds of fat

Calculating Lean Body Mass

To find the amount of you that is lean body mass (LBM), just rework the previous equation:

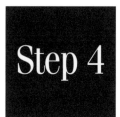

Figure out how much lean body mass you have.

> Current weight _____ (pounds) – fat _____ (pounds)
> = _____ pounds of lean body mass (LBM)

By figuring your lean body mass you now know exactly how much metabolically active (calorie-burning) tissue you have. This number is essential to many of the calculations we will do later. We can make an assumption that you want to keep all this lean body mass or even increase it a little while you lose the fat. After all, that is one of the main goals of *The Ultimate Lean Routine*!

Determining Your Goal Body Fat Percentage

Big question: What is a realistic loss in terms of body fat percentage over twelve weeks? Obviously, you could go for the gold and claim you want to lose half or more of your fat. However, in most cases this would not be realistic. As important as having a goal is having one that is actually achievable—one that you know you have a good chance of reaching. Here's what we have found works best: If you intend to be reasonably diligent about sticking to the program, you can use a multiplier of .85 against your current body fat percentage. If you intend to take it a step further and be aggressive about the program, you should use a multiplier of .80. And if you are ready to commit to being fanatical, and stick very closely to the program, you can use .75 as your multiplier.

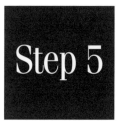

Establish your goal body fat.

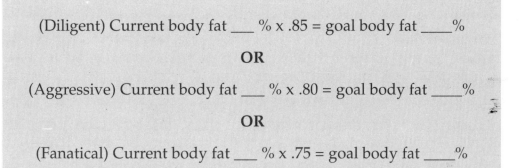

> (Diligent) Current body fat ___ % x .85 = goal body fat ____%
>
> **OR**
>
> (Aggressive) Current body fat ___ % x .80 = goal body fat ____%
>
> **OR**
>
> (Fanatical) Current body fat ___ % x .75 = goal body fat ____%

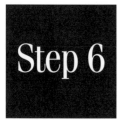

Step 6

Establish your goal body weight.

Determining Your Goal Weight
Based on LBM and Goal Body Fat

Obviously, if you intend to keep your LBM constant and decrease your percent of body fat, you will be at a new and lighter weight. Use the following formula to determine what that new, lighter goal weight will be:

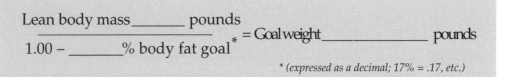

$$\frac{\text{Lean body mass}\underline{\qquad}\text{ pounds}}{1.00 - \underline{\qquad}\%\text{ body fat goal}^*} = \text{Goal weight}\underline{\qquad\qquad}\text{ pounds}$$

* *(expressed as a decimal; 17% = .17, etc.)*

Here is an example of the first six steps in action: Joe Average weighs in at 200 pounds and, with the calipers, determines that he is carrying 20% body fat. Twenty percent of 200 pounds is 40, so he knows he has 40 pounds of fat. He figures his lean body mass is 200 pounds – 40 pounds of fat = 160 pounds of lean body mass.

Joe decides he will be aggressive about his fat loss, so he multiplies his current body fat percentage of 20% by .80 and arrives at a realistic goal of 16% body fat. (It might not sound like a lot to lose but we'll soon see that this represents a 24% decrease in total fat in Joe's case.) Using the formula to determine Joe's goal weight, 160 (LBM) divided by (1.00 – .16) is the same as 160 ÷ .84 = 190.5 (rounding off). Therefore, assuming Joe does the workouts and eats right and doesn't lose any muscle tissue in the process, his goal weight will be 190.5 pounds, at which point he should be at or close to 16%body fat.

If that actually happens, how much fat will he have lost? Well, at 190.5 pounds and 16% body fat, Joe will have only 30.5 pounds of fat. Therefore, if he loses the 9.5 pounds of fat from the 40 he originally had, **he will have lost a total of 24% of all the fat on his body** (9.5 ÷ 40 = .2375 [rounded to .24]) ! And this is going from just 20% to 16% body fat. Is it possible to do that in twelve weeks on *The Ultimate Lean Routine*? Absolutely. In Joe's case, that's an average deficit of about 400 calories a day over the 12 weeks. As we will see shortly, some of that deficit comes from a slight dietary deficiency made up by burning stored fat in the workouts, some from increased metabolism throughout the rest of the day and some from a more fuel-efficient eating schedule. Of course, it doesn't come without hard work and discipline, but that's what helps provide. In this case, Joe will need to work up to burning 600 or 700 calories per workout by the end of the twelve weeks to accomplish his goal. The way the workouts are designed and scheduled, this should be very achievable by Joe or anyone else with similar starting abilities.

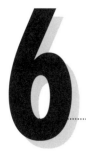

The IDEAL (Individually Designed Eating Agenda and Lifestyle) Diet

Now that we have learned about usage and storage of the three food fuels, and we know how much active calorie-burning tissue (LBM) we have, we can begin to formulate a precise plan for eating that will give us all the energy necessary to work out, to burn fat, and to otherwise function efficiently, without having to guess at it every day. After all, we wouldn't want to take in too much or too little fuel and, as a result, sabotage our fat loss plans. In this section we will be discussing an IDEAL diet. It is an *Individually Designed Eating Agenda and Lifestyle* based entirely on your specific requirements. This IDEAL diet should be used as a guideline for a lifestyle of eating. If you can follow it precisely, you will have maximum results over the twelve weeks. If you can't follow it precisely, just remember that coming close to the IDEAL as often as you can will still produce significant results. Going off the plan once in a while will not ruin your efforts as long as the overall effect is a diet and lifestyle trend that comes close to this IDEAL. Does this now mean that you will have to chart calories and grams for everything you eat over the next twelve weeks? Absolutely not. You will need to do some initial calculations to get a feel for your own requirements. Then, at the end of this chapter you will find a way to evaluate "intuitively" the kind of day you had diet-wise using a simple grading system. These are the only dietary numbers you will need to record in your logbook.

▼

To lose fat you have to burn off more calories than you take in.

Calories

In figuring basic energy requirements, it is necessary to use a common denominator for "energy units in" and "energy units out." That common denominator is the "calorie," a term with which most of us are all too familiar. Losing body fat can almost always be reduced to this equation: Burn more calories than you eat, and you'll lose fat. Of course, there are qualifications like avoiding extreme diets (remember the survival response and lowered metabolism that occur when calories in are *too* few) and not overtraining. It is important to be aware of both how much you are eating and how much fat-burning, muscle-building exercise you intend to do.

A review of the basic caloric contents of our three fuels yields the following numbers:

Fat = 9 calories per gram

Carbohydrate = 4 calories per gram

Protein = 4 calories per gram

The IDEAL Amounts of Fuel

Over the years, we've seen the health and fitness industries put forth many different ranges of dietary recommendations based on percentages of the three fuels. But formulas that call for ratios of x% calories from protein, x% from fat, and x% from carbs do not always take into consideration our varying individual differences in protein requirements, nor do they account for our different overall caloric requirements due to differences in lean body mass, sex, age, or lifestyle. Therefore, our first order of business must be to determine our exact individual and unique daily caloric requirements. Then, after we've determined our caloric requirements, we can each build our own unique eating plan using the IDEAL formula.

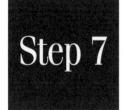

Step 7

Figure out how many calories your body needs each day.

Figuring Your Daily Caloric Requirements

Use this easy three-stage process to figure the exact number of calories you will need each day on :

1. First, determine your approximate resting metabolic requirement (RMR) in calories. Men should use a figure of 13 calories for each pound of lean body mass as you figured in Step 4 of Chapter 5. Women should use a figure of twelve calories for each pound of lean body mass. The total will give you your RMR, a figure equal to the bare minimum number of calories your body needs to maintain itself under conditions of little or no activity (sleeping, walking, sitting, etc.).

2. Next, apply a "lifestyle multiplier" which accounts for your general activity level throughout the day (not including your workout). You

simply multiply your RMR by this number. Although the following list may not contain your exact occupational workload, you should be able to match yours up fairly closely with the examples given:

light office work, mostly seated 1.2

housework, including shopping, errands 1.3

clerical, on feet most of the day doing light work 1.4

light construction or lots of walking 1.5

heavy construction, warehousing, moving, etc. 1.6

3. Finally, add to this a number equal to **one-half the total additional calories you will use during your average aerobic workout.** To do this accurately, you will have to refer to the stationary cycling section (Chapter 7) to determine exactly how many calories you will be burning during each workout. To give you some idea, depending on your current fitness level, the range should be from 150 (½ of 300 calories) at the low end, to 650 (½ of 1,300 calories) at the highest possible level for elite athletes. Most people starting this program will probably burn from 450 to 750 calories in the first workouts (which means they'd plug in half those numbers, or somewhere between 225 and 375 calories).

The total number determined by completing stages 1, 2 and 3 is the basis upon which you will "build" an eating plan for the next twelve weeks. This (and your stored fat!) should cover all your caloric needs throughout the day. This eating plan applies universally, regardless of your fat-loss goals. Loss of body fat will now occur as a result of:

1. a slight **daily caloric intake deficit**
2. **an increase in the calories burned during your aerobic workouts**
3. a strategic **change in the time of day you eat**
4. an **increase in resting metabolic rate** (fat burned at rest)

After the twelve weeks are up, you can refigure your caloric requirements to maintain your new body fat percentage based on the same equation, except you will add back the missing calories from stage 3 above that created your ongoing deficit. That is, instead of accounting for only half the calories you burned in your workout, you'll eventually account for all of them in your diet, sort of an extra eating reward for all your hard work.

Reviewing The Formula For Total Caloric Intake

1. LBM (lean body mass from Step 4 in Chapter 5)_____ pounds x 13 (men) or 12 (women) = _____ calories resting metabolic rate (RMR)

2. Multiply that RMR number by your lifestyle factor (1.2, 1.3, 1.4, 1.5, or 1.6 *[see chart]*) = _____ calories

3. Add in half the number of calories you will burn in your aerobic workout:

   RMR x lifestyle factor + half the calories burned working out = Total daily caloric intake every day over the 12 weeks

Now, here's an example of the plan at work:

From the calculations done earlier, Joe knows that he has 160 pounds of lean body mass. To determine his RMR (resting metabolic rate) he multiplies his lean body mass in pounds (160) times the RMR factor for men (13 calories per pound of lean body mass) to arrive at 160 x 13 = 2,080 calories per day RMR. Next, because Joe works at an office and sits around most of the day, he multiplies his RMR by his "lifestyle multiplier" to see how many calories he will burn when we adjust for normal daily activity. In this case it is 1.2, so 2,080 x 1.2 = 2,496. Finally, we add a number equal to one-half the total calories Joe will be burning during his average workout. Because Joe plans to burn an average 530 calories in each aerobic workout his first week (see Chapter 7), he will add half that number (or 265) to his total RMR x lifestyle multiplier: Therefore, 2,496 + 265 = 2,761 total calories needed per day.

The IDEAL Formula—
Determining Your Breakdown of Fats, Carbs and Protein

1. Calculate protein in the ratio of 1.0 grams protein to each pound of current lean body mass.

2. Calculate fats not to exceed 20% of total daily calories.

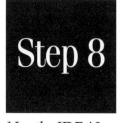

Step 8

Use the IDEAL formula to determine exactly how much protein, carbohydrate, and fat you need.

3. Calculate carbohydrates to make up the balance of total daily calories.

Now that you know what your daily caloric intake should be, you can use the IDEAL formula ratios to determine exactly how much protein, carbohydrate, and fat should comprise that diet. You will want to know not only how many calories each fuel represents, but also how many grams you should eat. Remember that this represents an IDEAL diet.

> 1. **PROTEIN REQUIREMENT:** _____ lean body mass in pounds x 1.0 = _____ grams of protein per day. To see how many calories this amount of protein would contribute to the total daily caloric requirement, take your figure _____ grams of protein per day (from preceding calculation) and multiply it by 4. So, _____ grams of protein per day x 4 calories per gram = _____ calories of protein per day. Now you know both the number of grams of protein you need (which you will find on most food packaging labels) as well as how many calories that amount of protein will contribute to the total daily caloric requirement.

In Joe's case, to determine his protein requirements, we multiply his lean body mass by 1.0 grams. So, his 160 pounds LBM x 1.0 grams of protein per pound = 112 grams of protein. Then, to get the number of calories that this amount of protein represents, we multiply 160 times 4 calories per gram to arrive at 640 calories from protein each day.

> 2. **FAT REQUIREMENT:** _____ total daily caloric requirement x 20% = _____ calories from fat allowed each day. Then, to find out exactly how many grams of fat that equals, we divide the number of calories from fat allowed each day by 9 calories per gram. So, _____ calories from fat ÷ 9 calories per gram = _____ grams of fat allowed each day. Knowing both these numbers, we can check labels for "fat grams" to keep on track, and we also know just how many calories that amount of fat is contributing to our total daily caloric requirement.

As for Joe, to determine his fat "allowance," we multiply the 2,761 total calories we know he'll be eating by 20% to get 552 calories from fat. Then, in terms of grams, we divide 552 by 9 calories per gram to arrive at 61 grams of fat per day.

> 3. **CARBOHYDRATE REQUIREMENT:** _____ total daily caloric requirement – (_____ daily fat calories + _____ daily protein calories) = _____ daily carbohydrate calories. Then, to find out how many grams of carbohydrate this represents (because we'll read grams of carbohydrate on all labels), we divide that number by 4 calories per gram: So, _____ daily carbohydrate calories ÷ 4 calories per gram = _____ grams of carbohydrate each day.

Back to Joe once again, to determine carbohydrate intake we just add protein calories to fat calories and then subtract that number from his daily total calorie allowance of 2,761. In this case, 552 daily fat calories plus 640 daily protein calories add up to 1,192, which we will then subtract from 2,761 total daily calories to leave a balance of 1,569 calories from carbohydrate. In terms of grams of carbs, that would be: 1,569 ÷ 4 calories per gram = 392 grams of carbohydrate. Now Joe knows exactly how much of each fuel he needs to eat each day:

> **Joe's IDEAL Fuel Breakdown per Day:**
>
> Protein . . . . .160 grams . . . . .640 calories
> Fat .61 grams . . . . .552 calories
> Carbohydrates . . . . .392 grams . . . . .1,569 calories
> **Total Calories** . . . .**2,761 calories**

Joe's overall breakdown of proteins/fats/carbs on a percentage basis is protein, 231/2; fats, 20%; and carbs, 57. This of course, will be individualized to your lean body mass variable.

Note: Food labels and food reference books often indicate exactly how much protein, fat and carbs are in a given serving. Usually these labels will give you both weight in grams and caloric value for each fuel. However, since occasionally these labels will refer to grams only and other times refer to calories only, it is important to know how to figure your amounts both ways (see later information on reading labels).

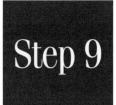

Step 9

Calculate when to eat what.

Figuring Out How Much to Eat and When

There is one more important principle to follow in building the IDEAL diet. Now that you know exactly what to eat during each day, you need to know when or how often throughout the day to eat. Otherwise your fuel intake, even if perfect in the amounts of calories and breakdown of components, could work against you. The IDEAL schedule here is also quite simple:

- Eat **30%** of your calories between the time you get up and 10:00 a.m.

- Eat the **next 40%** of your calories after 10:00 a.m. but before 3:00 p.m.

- Eat the **balance of your calories** (the remaining 30%) between 3:00 p.m. and 8:00 p.m.

Keep the mix of fat/carb/protein relatively similar throughout the day. Now that you know how much protein/fats/carbs to eat in a day, spread out the portions evenly so each meal has a balance of the three.

THE 30/40/30 IDEAL SCHEDULE

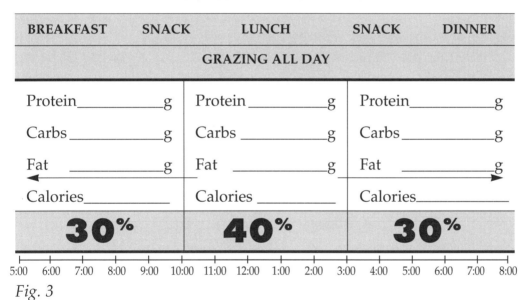

Fig. 3

In the best of all possible worlds, eating three small meals a day with a small snack between each is the best way to eat, as long as you can stick to the IDEAL formula for the amount of foods and the timing of your eating. Nutritionists refer to this form of eating as "grazing." However, in the real world, grazing sometimes just isn't practical due to work schedules or other factors. In this case the most important considerations are:

1.

EAT A HEALTHY BREAKFAST.

Oatmeal, egg whites, toast, bagels, fresh fruit;
low-sugar, high-fiber cereal with nonfat milk

2.

EAT A SUBSTANTIAL MIDDAY MEAL.

Skinless chicken breast, grilled fish, tuna or turkey sandwich, large
green salad with low-fat dressing, pasta with low-fat sauce, low-fat soups,
steamed vegetables, rice, baked potatoes, lentils, beans, bread

3.

EAT HEALTHY SNACKS.

Following the "grazing" principle, it is best to spread your calories over a longer
time span, so that your meals are smaller. I recommend using a protein powder
drink, or other choices such as rice cakes, carrots, raw
vegetables, fruit, salsa and nonfat chips, hot-air popcorn, nonfat yogurt.

4.

EAT A SMALL EVENING MEAL.

Similar to your midday meal selections, only smaller portions or
a larger percentage of salad and steamed vegetables

▼

Eating all the correct things but doing so at the wrong times of day will sabotage your program.

Your eating schedule is critical to your success in *The Ultimate Lean Routine*. Imagine, for example, if we ate all of our daily allotment of food—even a perfect breakdown of calories, protein, fats, and carbs—at one big meal at nine o'clock each night. Don't laugh. There are actually people who do this sort of thing and then wonder why they can't seem to shed the pounds! Well, here's what would happen to that meal: All of the fat, most of the carbohydrate, and some of the protein would be converted to stored fat as we slept that night with a gut full of food. Upon our waking the next morning and not eating breakfast, our blood sugar would start off relatively low and begin a slow descent throughout the day, making us cranky and sleepy and preventing us from working effectively. Our workout would suffer even more as our liver and muscle glycogen reserves were quickly depleted from a day of being squandered to boost brain fuel. Our precious lean body mass would slowly shrink as protein was also called upon (*sacrificed* is more like it) for use as fuel in the absence of a regular supply of glucose. Our basal metabolic rate would begin to slow with this reduction in LBM. By the time 9 p.m. (dinnertime) rolled around the next night, this process of fat storage and muscle atrophy would begin all over as even more fuel was converted to fat while we slept, and so on, all the while making us fatter and weaker. As you can see, this worst case scenario demonstrates that even if your diet is perfect in composition, it is still possible to sabotage your goals by eating at the wrong times of day.

Remember that our intent is to use food as fuel to get us through the day with energy and to work **for** us in burning off that fat. Eating 30% of your calories earlier in the day in the form of a healthy breakfast, and possibly even including a midmorning snack in that 30%, primes the fuel pump for a day of greater energy. We burn off almost 100 grams of stored glycogen during our night's sleep. This is because even while we sleep, the brain is still "working" and it runs only on glucose, which it gets by taking glycogen out of storage. As a result, we often wake up slightly glycogen-depleted. Making certain we get 80 to 100 grams of carbohydrate into us first thing—along with some protein and a little fat to minimize any dramatic insulin effect—ensures that most of that carbohydrate will be used to raise blood glucose and to restore glycogen supplies. This fuel-efficient way of beginning the day is important regardless of when we choose to do workouts, but it is absolutely **critical** if we work out in the morning. And, although it is preferable to eat before your workout, if you are unable to do so before a very early morning workout, then try to eat at least something—anything—beforehand and follow it soon after your workout (and definitely before 10:00 a.m.) with the rest of the morning's 30%.

The next 40% of your total calories should be consumed during the midday segment. Because the body's metabolic processes are most active at this time, more fuel is required for maintaining energy reserves between 10:00 a.m. and 3:00 p.m. This is also generally the most convenient time of day to focus on obtaining your protein requirements. Therefore, if you've chosen to include chicken, fish or red meat in your eating plan (in modest amounts, of course), this would be the best time of day to eat them, along with appropriate amounts of fat and carbohydrate to balance out the calories.

▼

Taking in 40% of calories during the middle part of the day takes advantage of the body's elevated metabolic rate at that time.

The Evening Meal

Regardless of when you work out, you should never eat a large meal at the end of the day. As in our "worst case scenario," one of the biggest mistakes we can make is to have our biggest meal in the evening. Many of us view this as a "reward" for a long day at work or for a supertough workout. But the fact is that consuming 50%, 60%, or in many cases even 70% of our total daily calories in a four-course evening meal leaves us with a gut full of fuel and no place to burn it. As in the graphic example given previously, much of that fuel—beyond maybe 100 grams of carbohydrate that will be used to replace glycogen—simply gets converted to fat while we sleep. As we've each experienced, after any fuel is stored as

▼

Avoid eating large evening meals. If you feel that you must fill up, eat extra steamed vegetables or a large salad.

fat, it becomes at least fifty times harder to get back out of fat-storage. Of course, this is completely counterproductive to the fat *burning* purpose of *The Ultimate Lean Routine*. Therefore, always make your evening meal relatively light, not exceeding 30% of your day's total calories. One way to continue to give yourself that feeling of "reward" is to make the evening meal filling yet healthy, as in the form of a large salad, baked potatoes or steamed vegetables with rice. Provided you stay away from high-fat salad dressings or butter on the vegetables, you can eat just about all you want and still have that feeling of fullness without exceeding your caloric budget. Small amounts of meat, fish, tofu, or beans can be added for flavor and to contribute protein without pushing calories over the limit. If you crave something sweet at the end of the day, treat yourself to fresh fruit, or, provided you are within your caloric parameters, have a frozen non-fat dessert.

Finally, it is also counterproductive to go to bed hungry. The message of starvation is sent to the working brain throughout the night, which further slows down your resting metabolic rate. A light meal of the right proportion best ensures a productive fat burning night.

Let's go back to Joe, who is now figuring the schedule for his IDEAL diet. Joe will want to break down his day as follows:

2,761 (daily total) x 30% = 828 calories before 10 a.m.

2,761 x 40% = 1,105 between 10 a.m. and 3 p.m.

2,761 x 30% = 828 between 3 p.m. and bedtime
(preferably before 8 p.m.).

JOE'S 30/40/30% IDEAL SCHEDULE

BREAKFAST	SNACK	LUNCH		SNACK	DINNER
←		GRAZING ALL DAY			→
Protein	33 g	Protein	46 g	Protein	33 g
Carbs	132 g	Carbs	176 g	Carbs	132 g
Fat	18 g	Fat	25 g	Fat	18 g
Calories	828	Calories	1105	Calories	828
30%		**40%**		**30%**	

5:00 6:00 7:00 8:00 9:00 10:00 11:00 12:00 1:00 2:00 3:00 4:00 5:00 6:00 7:00 8:00

Fig. 3

Additionally, Joe will try to further divide up the components of his diet along the same 30/40/30% schedule, so that he has 30% of his protein, 30% of his carbs, and 30% of his fat in the morning, 40% of each in the midday, and 30% at the end of the day. He knows from Step 8 exactly what his daily totals are; now all he needs to do is take 30%, 40%, and 30% of each to fill in the blanks.

The Secret to Topping off the Fuel Tank

In order to be best prepared for your next workout, one of the smartest things you can do is to consume 80 to 100 grams of carbohydrate immediately after every workout. These *Ultimate Lean Routine* workouts will definitely deplete some of your glycogen reserves, so it will always be necessary to "top them off" before beginning the next workout. Of course, you can do this by simply eating according to your regular schedule as we just outlined, because the body is always gradually rebuilding glycogen reserves, but here's a little secret: Exercise physiology research has shown that 80 to 100 grams of carbohydrate taken within forty-five minutes of the completion of a workout speed up the glycogen-rebuilding process and lead to faster recovery and a better starting point for the next day's workout. Throwing protein (20-30 grams) into the equation seems to help as well. Some excellent postworkout drinks containing the right blend of carbohydrate and protein can now be found in most health food stores. Topping off the tank this way after every workout also ensures that those calories will not be stored as fat. This is true whether you are doing early, midday or even late workouts. Of course, you have to account for these calories and grams like any others in your 30/40/30% strategy, but it should be easy to fit these 300 to 400 important calories into your eating plan without going over the limits.

▼

Top off your fuel tank immediately after each workout.

A Quick Note on Your Choice of Food

As a general rule of thumb, try to choose the foods that are as close to their natural sources or as "close to the farm" as possible. Try not to eat out of wrappers, plastic, boxes, or cans. Instead choose fresh vegetables, grains, fruits, poultry, fish, and nonfat dairy. Processed foods tend to be filled with preservatives and high levels of sodium. The cooking in processing tends to rob the foods of their organic nutrients and change their natural properties. Often, food that is processed has also been stripped of its fiber, which is responsible for maintaining an efficient digestive system. Some people view the use of preservatives in many processed foods as merely pollutants to your system, altering the way your system deals with food.

A Quick Note on Salt

▼

Medical research has shown that excessive salt can be responsible for high blood pressure, strokes, kidney failure and hypertension.

A general rule of thumb is to keep your salt intake under 2,000 mg a day (about 1 teaspoon). Even if you don't use a salt shaker, you should still pay attention. Sodium is present in significant amounts in much of the grocery foods, fast foods and restaurant foods, and is often hiding in "healthy" foods as well. Over time, the American palate has grown accustomed to the flavor that salt brings to food, and in general, we take in far too much salt. Medical research has shown that excessive salt can be responsible for high blood pressure, strokes, kidney failure and hypertension. Also, salt causes fluid retention, which is definitely not a "lean" quality. Remember that mustard, pickles, salad dressings, breakfast cereals and snacks can be high in sodium. Read your labels and police your salt intake.

A Quick Note on Vitamins

Vitamins are micronutrients that have no caloric value. However, they are essential to life and absolutely critical to the production of energy. Just as fat, protein and carbohydrate are the fuels we burn, vitamins are the "spark plugs" that help us burn these fuels. Over the past decade much research has been done on vitamins and their contributions to health and to fitness. The jury is still out on whether or not supplementing your diet with vitamins can make a significant difference in fat metabolism and muscle growth, but the evidence is very strong that taking higher amounts of certain vitamins, especially the antioxidant vitamins C, E, and beta carotene, can dramatically lower your risks of cancer and heart disease. If you are sticking to the IDEAL plan outlined previously, chances are that your diet is providing a fair amount of these micronutrient vitamins and minerals. This will be particularly true for anyone getting most of their fuel from fruits, vegetables, and whole grains. Still, there is evidence that taking in extra amounts of certain antioxidant vitamins and minerals can enhance your training and possibly help prevent injury. It is also important for women to take in 800-1,500 mg of calcium daily. Low levels of calcium can be responsible for low bone density and premature osteoporosis. Iron is another mineral important for active women and most men. Low levels of iron can sabotage overall energy levels throughout the day and during your workouts and can ultimately lead to anemia. Therefore, it is recommended that you take a daily multi-vitamin supplement. Look for one that is in the form of a powder-filled capsule rather than a tablet. Capsules dissolve much more easily and are absorbed more readily than rock-hard tablets. Also, look for one that provides amounts of nutrients at or slightly higher than 100% of the RDA. Finally, always take your vitamin supplements with a meal to ensure optimal absorption.

A Quick Note on Types of Fat

While we have been discussing the necessity to cut back on total fat intake, there are some differences in types of dietary fat. Certain fats are now considered by the medical and health community to be "better" than other types of fats. Several are even believed to be therapeutic for some people with high cholesterol and heart disease. Recent investigations indicate that, in general, **naturally derived fats are better for you than processed fats.** Food processors often "hydrogenate" certain fats to give them more stability or allow them to become semisolid at room temperature. Stick margarine is an example of one such common hydrogenated product. The problem with processed fats is that they become higher in "transfatty acids," which have been shown to cause cholesterol buildup and play a role in other degenerative processes. On the other hand, most naturally derived fats, whether poly- or mono-unsaturated (and whether animal or plant), have functions that contribute to normal cell wall construction and other processes more suitable to life. If we consider evolution and our survival adaptations once more, it makes sense that any fats developed in the laboratory in modern times (like processed fats) would have a more adverse effect on us than those natural fats we have adapted to and survived on quite suitably for millions of years.

▼

Avoid hydrogenated processed fats, which are high in transfatty acids.

As a general rule of thumb, almost all the fat in grains and vegetables is "safe." The only exception is palm-kernel oil. Stay away from it whenever possible. Otherwise, cold-pressed oils such as olive, safflower, and canola are considered to be beneficial when consumed in moderation. Look for salad dressings using those oils instead of other more processed oils. Avoid animal and dairy fats whenever possible. Buy lean cuts of meat or skinless chicken, and use only 1% or nonfat milk.

Ultimately, if you are being diligent about your eating program and keeping your total fat "allowance" at or below 20% of calories, you are probably eating healthy enough that the amount of unhealthy fat in your diet will be at an acceptable level.

A Quick Note on Water

▼

Water intake is extremely important. Try to drink at least eight cups a day.

Water is essential for human life. Over 70% of the human body consists of water. Muscles are actually closer to 85% water. Athletes and other fit individuals depend on water to cool themselves (through sweat) and to help eliminate toxins. Water helps us metabolize fats easier. Virtually all chemical reactions occurring in the body require water. Without water, humans are able to exist for only a few days before facing life-threatening consequences. Clearly, then, water intake is an important part of one's daily maintenance, and anyone would be well advised to take in eight (or more) cups a day. Luckily, much of the food we eat, especially fruits and vegetables, is high in water content, so we don't necessarily need to spend all our time at the water cooler. Juices, teas, soups, and other forms of liquid (except alcohol) count also. Nevertheless, it is important to pay attention to the amount of water we are drinking and make an effort to take in eight cups or the equivalent.

Is Meat Protein Better Than Plant Protein?

Many people are under the impression that protein from meat is of a higher quality than protein from plant sources. It's not. Amino acids are amino acids, whether they come from plants or animals. The real question is whether we are getting all twenty-two possible amino acids in our diet. Although humans are able to recycle many of the twenty-two amino acids that comprise protein, there are eight amino acids we are unable to remanufacture. These eight have become known as "essential" amino acids because getting them in our diet is essential to health. Whereas most animal protein contains all twenty-two amino acids in various amounts, most plant sources are somewhat incomplete, each plant having fewer than all twenty-two amino acids in differing amounts. Still, within the plant kingdom, all twenty-two amino acids can be accounted for quite easily by combining different grains, fruits and vegetables. As long as you are getting all twenty-two amino acids from one source or another, and particularly the eight "essential" amino acids, your body won't care whether they come from animal or vegetable sources.

The main benefit to a diet that includes meat, chicken, and fish is that your requirements for complete protein can be met quite easily. The drawback is that animal protein sources also tend to be higher in fat. However, by trimming off visible fat, eliminating skin, broiling instead of frying, and eating smaller portions, you can get ample amounts of protein while keeping your fat intake low.

On the other hand, some people feel that a vegetarian diet is not only a legitimate source of high quality protein, but also a healthier alternative, because plant sources are almost always lower in fat, except for certain protein-rich foods like nuts, seeds, avocados and some types of tofu. Just be certain not only that you are obtaining your total daily protein requirements, but also that all essential amino acids are accounted for. The best way for vegetarians to ensure this is to regularly include beans, lentils, peas, and other legumes in the diet. These supply certain amino acids absent in grains, fruits, and leafy vegetables, and, when eaten in combination, make complete proteins.

The bottom line is that it is possible to eat healthy either way as long as you are paying attention to what is in the foods you eat. The best way to do this is by reading and understanding the food labels.

Hints on Reading the Labels

As of 1994, all packaged food is required to have nutritional information labeling that conforms to a standard established by the Food and Drug Administration. Reading the "nutrition fact" label is the easiest way to get a handle on exactly what's in the food you are eating. The sample on page 45 *(Fig. 5)* lists examples of what you might find on a label and how to decipher that information.

a. New labels have fairly realistic estimations of "serving size." Whether or not you consider the portion or amount per serving appropriate for you, keep in mind that the rest of the label contains information relative only to this listed serving size or portion, not necessarily the whole bag, box, or can. Therefore, if you intend to eat double or triple (or half) the listed serving size, be sure to double or triple (or halve) all the other numbers on the label.

b. "Calories" per serving should be self-explanatory. More important once again is calories from fat. To determine exactly how "fat-free" or fat-laden each serving is, divide "calories from fat" by total calories and multiply by 100 to get "percent calories from fat." If it is less than 30%, you should be OK provided you are eating substantial amounts of complex

▼

Vegetarians need to be extra diligent in seeking higher quality sources of protein.

▼

Most of what you need to know about the foods you're eating can be found on the nutrition fact label.

carbohydrate-rich foods (which will, almost by definition, be very low in fat). And even if this particular product contains fat in an amount higher than 30%, your main goal number is still total fat grams per day.

c. "% Daily Value" is a general reference guide based on an assumed daily calorie intake of 2,000 and the government's recommendation that 30% of your calories come from fat (remember, we're at 20%) and 60% carbs (our number is the remaining balance of protein and carbs). Your number will probably be different, so just note that all the numbers in this column express a percentage of that theoretical 2,000 calorie, 60/30/10% diet, and not the *Ultimate Lean Routine* breakdown.

d. Obviously, the big number everyone is concerned with is fat, and all labels get this news out of the way first. Total fat grams is what we are most interested in tracking, so pay close attention to this one. As for the saturated/unsaturated breakdown, as was mentioned before, if your total fat intake is under control and your are eating mostly unprocessed foods, you should be OK.

e. "Total Carbohydrate" is the main number to seek out in this category. Higher dietary fiber is considered good, a low number for "Sugar" is also considered good, because this refers to simple sugars. Assume that most of whatever is not sugars will be complex carbs. Remember that we are looking to get a handle on grams per day.

f. "Protein," expressed in grams per serving, ought to be self-explanatory. Remember, though, this won't identify the amino acid breakdown of your protein, just total grams per day.

g. "Vitamin" content is expressed only as a percent of the RDA. Note whether your food is "nutritious" beyond just the three fuels.

h. This area has nothing to do with what's inside. It is a reference guide for the consumer to see what the government's recommendations for an average 2,000-calorie or 2,500-calorie diet should be. By now, you already know about 1,000% more than the average consumer, so disregard these numbers and use your own IDEAL calculations.

i. The "Ingredients" are listed in a descending order of quantity. New labels are required to list ingredients more specifically than in the past. This may assist you in identifying foods that contain artificial ingredients, colorings, additives, and preservatives—so you can avoid them, obviously.

Fig. 5

Nutrition Facts

Serving Size 1/2 cup (140g) Cooked
Servings Per Container 12

a.

Amount Per Serving

b.

Calories 170   Calories from Fat 25

% Daily Value*

c.

d.

Total Fat 3g	**5**%
Saturated Fat 0g	**0**%
Cholesterol 0mg	**0**%
Sodium 15mg	**1**%
Total Carbohydrate 30g	**10**%
Dietary Fiber 6g	**24**%
Sugars 0g	
Protein 6g	

e.

f.

Vitamin A 0%	•	Vitamin C 0%
Calcium 2%	•	Iron 8%

g.

*Percent Daily Values are based on a 2,000 calorie diet. Your daily values may be higher or lower depending on your calorie needs:

	Calories	2,000	2,500
Total Fat	Less than	65g	80g
Sat Fat	Less than	20g	25g
Cholesterol	Less than	300mg	300mg
Sodium	Less than	2,400mg	2,400mg
Total Carbohydrate		300g	375g
Dietary Fiber		25g	30g

h.

Calories per gram:
Fat 9 • Carbohydrates 4 • Protein 4

INGREDIENTS: Whole Oats, Long Grain Brown Rice, Whole Rye, Whole Hard Red Winter Wheat, Whole Triticale, Whole Buckwheat, Whole Barley, Sesame Seeds.

i.

Keeping Track

▼

Develop an "instinctive" feel for how well you eat.

Now that you know so much about your diet, you may be asking how will you ever be able to keep track of it without writing everything down? It's easy, after you have completed your outline of how many calories and grams you need daily. Just give yourself a **score** at the end of each day which reflects *instinctively* how well you did in each category, and then add the five category scores up to arrive at one total score for the day. You may need to actually chart everything for the first few days to see how much of everything you actually do eat, but eventually you will begin to know how well (or not) you are doing without the burdensome task of tracking everything gram by gram. You may also begin to develop a pattern of meal choices that becomes easy to remember and fix each day. This is not to say that you need to eat the same things every day, but having a few breakfast choices, a selection of midday meals, a variety of healthy snacks, and a salad or steamed vegetable routine for dinner can make eating pleasurable, sensible and a breeze to track. Remember, **it is the understanding and awareness of a lean eating "style" that are most important.** Here's how it works:

For purposes of recording progress in your logbook, you will simply rate your whole day's fuel consumption on a scale of 5 to 1 for each of the five categories, with 5 being right on target (your IDEAL) and 1 being completely "off target." Notice that we don't count calories. That's because your fat, protein and carbohydrate gram numbers will automatically account for calories. Also, because the timing of your eating is crucial, you get double points in that category. These are the only numbers you will need to record:

Fig. 6

IDEAL Diet Evaluation

	IDEAL				Off Target		
Water Intake	5	4	3	2	1		+
Fat Intake	5	4	3	2	1		+
Protein Intake	5	4	3	2	1		+
Carb Intake	5	4	3	2	1		+
30/40/30%	10	8	6	4	0		=
					TOTAL SCORE		

25–30 = excellent; 19–24 = good; 18 or less = needs work

KEY

Total water intake: If you hit your IDEAL number of eight glasses for the day, give yourself a 5 here. Six or seven glasses, give yourself a 4. Four or five glasses ranks a 3. Give yourself a 2 if you drank only three glasses. A "camel day" of two or less rates only a 1.

Total fat intake: If you hit your IDEAL number of fat grams or were less than 5 grams over for the day, or any number under, give yourself a 5. Over by 10 to 15 grams give yourself a 4. Twenty to thirty grams too much and you get a 3. Forty to fifty over rates a 2. And anything over 50 beyond your target gets only a 1.

Total protein intake: Again, you get a 5 for being at or very close to your IDEAL number of grams of protein. Circle 4 if you came within 5-20 grams either way (too much is as undesirable as too little). Circle 3 if you were 20-30 grams off. Circle 2 if you were over 30 off. If you really messed up or fasted, circle 1.

Total carb intake: same idea. If you are right on target at your IDEAL number, or within 5%, give yourself a 5. Off by 5-10% either way, circle 4. Ten-twenty percent off, circle 3. Twenty-fifty percent off deserves only a 2, and way off track a 1.

30/40/30 schedule: This counts for twice the score, since timing is doubly important to the program. *Regardless* of how much you ate, if you divided it up the IDEAL 30/40/30% or within 5%, circle 10. Off by 5-10 % either way, circle 8. If any one part of the day was way off, but you still ate something during the other one or two segments, give yourself a 6. Say you skipped dinner, but had a large brunch or lunch, take a 4. If you fasted all day or if you gorged a late night meal, give yourself a 0.

After assigning a score to each category, simply add up the total of all five to arrive at one total score for the day. This is the barometer for how well you are doing on a day-to-day basis. Obviously, 30 would be a perfect score. Anything between 25 and 30 is excellent, between 19 and 24 is good but needs a little more work. Less than 18 will indicate that you need a lot more work to get the kind of results you are expecting.

Back to Joe, who has started tracking his meals. Let's look at one of his typical days. Joe drinks plenty of water every day, so he gives himself a perfect 5 for **water intake**. On this particular day, he figures his **fat intake** was over only by 15 grams, due mostly to an extra-oily pasta he had for lunch, so he records a 4. His **protein** intake was a little low overall because he was focusing on the complex carbs. He figures he's off by about 30 grams, so he gives himself a 3. No question in his mind, his **carb intake** was right on for the day, so that warrants another 5. Finally, he was a little light on the breakfast and didn't make it up with a snack before 10 a.m., while he also had a larger-than-planned evening meal, so he'll give himself an 8 under **30/40/30%**. His total for the day, at 25, is just inside the excellent standard. The entire procedure takes less than a minute, because, after spending some time learning about what's in the foods he eats, he's confident he can intuitively grade his performance without referring to charts and graphs anymore.

Fig. 7

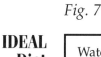

IDEAL Diet Evaluation

IDEAL ← → Off Target						
Water Intake	⑤	4	3	2	1	5	+
Fat Intake	5	④	3	2	1	4	+
Protein Intake	5	4	③	2	1	3	+
Carb Intake	⑤	4	3	2	1	5	+
30/40/30%	10	⑧	6	4	0	8	=
				TOTAL SCORE		25

25–30 = excellent; 19–24 = good; 18 or less = needs work

Four Big Fat Lies

Armed with new information on training and diet, it's time to take a look at the four big myths that the fitness industry has tried to sell us over the years and see how our new understanding of fuel consumption and fuel usage changes our approach:

1. One of the biggest myths in the diet and exercise world is that low-intensity prolonged exercise is the most effective way to burn fat. It's not. We now know that the most effective way to burn all fuel (and to lose fat for good) is to burn as many calories as you can in the time you have allotted to work out by doing moderately intense exercise. In fact, advanced fitness enthusiasts will often do very intense exercise. In other words, it's not the **type** of calories you burn during your workout (fat vs. carbohydrate), but plain and simply the **quantity** of calories. The faster or harder you go for a given period of time, the

more calories you burn and the more fat you lose. Given the choice between powerwalking three miles in one hour or running four and a half miles in forty minutes, the forty-minute run will result in a greater loss of fat because you'll burn 50% more calories (300 total for the walk and 450 total for the run). And it will take less time to accomplish. You'll also burn off more fat calories over the next several hours as you rest. **Never lose sight of your goal: It's not just how much fat you burn during a workout, it's how much you ultimately lose that counts.**

▼

It's a myth that low-intensity exercise is the best way to burn fat. Higher intensity exercise can burn more fat in less time.

2. The second major misconception people have is that, in order to lose fat we have to drastically reduce the amount of food we eat. In reality, **drastic** reductions in calories can cause us to retain fat by stimulating the **starvation survival response!** One of the basic human survival adaptations we discussed earlier occurs when radical reductions in caloric intake cause the body to conserve fat and to actually burn up muscle protein for energy—the most counterproductive thing we could possibly do! We have to eat in order to survive and in order to have enough energy to work out. It takes energy to burn fat! Most important are what types of food we eat and when we eat them.

3. The third common misconception is that only aerobic exercise can stimulate fat loss. Again the truth is that because only muscle and other lean body mass can burn fat, **the more muscle you have, the more fat you can burn both during exercise and at rest** (remember that at rest, muscle tissue derives 75%-90% of its energy from fats!). Any fat-loss program that emphasizes only aerobic activity will likely result in loss of some of this precious muscle tissue, too (which is why running, by itself an effective way to lose weight in the forms of both fat and muscle, is not the most effective way to lose just fat). Weight training and certain other forms of anaerobic cross-training actually help preserve or build lean muscle, leaving you looking better and more toned and defined as well as having more strength to complete every workout.

4. The fourth misconception is that if you don't eat fat, you won't store fat. The truth is: The bottom line in weight loss is calories in vs. calories out, regardless of the type of calories consumed. There is a tendency for people to overeat nonfat foods and desserts because they think those nonfat treats can't be converted and stored as fat. They can—and will—if you have exceeded your daily caloric requirement.

▼

It's a myth that nonfat foods can't make you fat. The bottom line in weight loss is calories in vs. calories out.

However, there is a further distinction worth discussing if you do consume extra calories. Excess carbohydrate or protein calories require the body to burn 27% of the actual calories to convert them to stored fat, whereas fat calories require only 3%. In other words, if you eat 500 calories of a carbohydrate or protein, 135 calories are burned in the storage process, leaving a net caloric intake of 365 extra calories. On the other hand, with 500 calories of fat, the body is able to store it as fat using only 15 calories, leaving 485 calories net. Excess calories are stored mostly as fat, regardless of the source, but carbohydrates and proteins are substantially "discounted" in the conversion process.

So exactly which exercises provide the right blend of both aerobic and anaerobic fat-burning body-sculpting results? The workouts described in the next chapter of *The Ultimate Lean Routine*, of course.

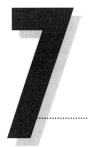

The Ultimate Lean Routine Workouts

The Ultimate Lean Routine Week by Week

The foundation of *The Ultimate Lean Routine* is a simple rotation of three uniquely complementary cross-training workouts designed to burn fat, build muscle and prevent injury. This rotation allows for the optimal rest of each working muscle, and fat-burning system between workouts.

Day 1: Stationary bicycling forty-five minutes to an hour

Day 2: Running/powerwalking/stairclimbing forty-five minutes to an hour

Day 3: Strength training with weights (ten exercises covering all major body parts) one hour

Day 4: Stationary bicycling up to an hour

Day 5: Running/powerwalking/stairclimbing up to an hour

Day 6: Strength training with weights (ten exercises) one hour

Day 7: Rest and recovery—day off

This cycle is repeated each week for twelve weeks as we progressively add resistance to each exercise over time. This holds true for both the aerobic workouts as well as the strength workouts. Your exact progress should be measured for each of the twenty-four workouts in each of the three cross-training disciplines. By recording this information in your logbook, you can keep exact track of your progress toward your goal daily and weekly, and from start to finish.

▼

It is never necessary to exceed sixty minutes in any of The Ultimate Lean Routine workouts.

Days 1 and 4: Stationary Cycling

Choosing Your Weapon

Although many other impressive equipment choices can be found in the gym, the stationary bike (also known as a "cycling ergometer") is still one of the most effective forms of aerobic activities available. Among the many benefits: They are almost universally available at gyms throughout the country; they are adaptable to anyone's size, shape or current level of fitness; they give anyone the ability to increase or decrease resistance incrementally from beginner level to world class; and their use can help you avoid injury. Most gyms have several brands and models of cycling ergometers, but whichever brand or model you use, be sure it has a "total calories used" feature. As you will see shortly, this is vital to our ability to **measure precisely the amount of work done each cycling day.** Also, if it's possible for you to do so, use the same bike each time you do these workouts. Stationary bicycle manufacturers often calibrate their bikes slightly differently. Therefore, in order to accurately compare your last ride to your next ride, it helps to stay on the same equipment.

Setting up the Bike Properly

First, set the seat height at a level that enables you to get almost a full leg extension. *(Photo 3)*

This fuller extension involves the largest number of leg muscle fibers and tends to lengthen them. It also involves more of the back of the upper thigh and butt—muscle groups that just about everyone wants to see taut and firm. Don't put the seat so high that you have to point your toes to reach the pedals or rock your hips back and forth to complete each revolution, both of which are clear indi-

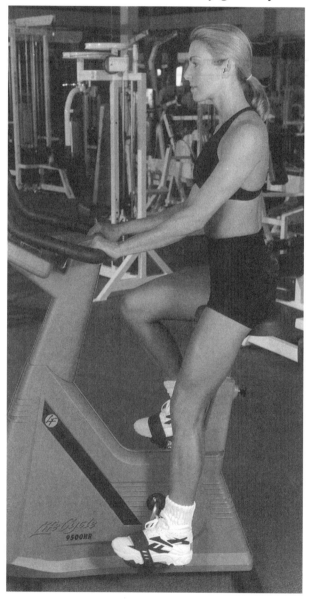

Photo 3

cations that the seat is too high. Conversely, if the seat is too low, you'll work a much smaller group of muscles and you will tend to overdevelop the quads and not work the butt and backs of the thighs enough.

Be sure the toeclip allows for a snug fit of your foot on the pedal so that the ball of your foot is over the center of the pedal. *(Photo 4)*

Again, not so tight that you cut off circulation. Record both these settings in your logbook for future reference.

Find a comfortable riding position either sitting upright or resting your arms on the handlebars as shown. *(Photo 5)*

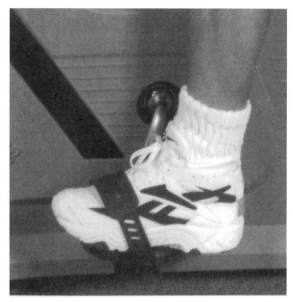

Photo 4

The Warm-Up

Begin pedaling and hit the start button. Select the manual mode on any bike, as opposed to one of the random or preprogrammed hill profiles. This way, you can control the entire workout yourself. Start with an easy warm-up on Level 1 or 2 for a few minutes. If you are a stronger rider and need a higher level to warm up, do so, but after anywhere from five to ten minutes of warm-up, go right into the work of this session. *(Photo 6)*

The Work Session

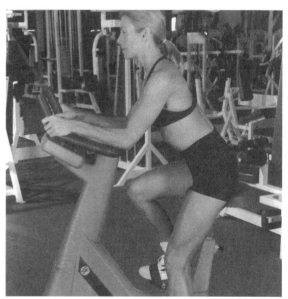

Photo 5

For starters, during your first few workouts it is important to find a resistance level that you can ride at steadily for thirty minutes without getting overly winded or having to stop. After your warm-up, **your primary mission will always be to burn as many calories as you can while staying within your lean training zone heart rate as outlined in the following sections.** Unlike in conventional fat-burning programs, **our goal in this program is to eventually maintain a steady heart rate and work out at the higher end of your lean training zone** (as opposed to the lower end of your "aerobic range"). As your fitness increases (not to mention your calorie-burning ability) you will find yourself able to go to a higher effort

▼

The goal is clear: Burn as many calories as you can in any given aerobic workout —as long as you don't exceed your lean training zone heart rate range.

level on the bike while still keeping within the upper end of your lean training zone, a true indication of aerobic efficiency and overall fitness.

The Lean Training Zone Heart Rates

The lean training zone represents the range of your heart rates, from the high end to the low end, within which you will burn the most calories for the time you spend training, without having to stop and rest.

Most other fitness programs have you figure all the work you will eventually do based on first determining your maximum heart rate. But maximum heart rates of people the same age can still vary tremendously from one individual to the next, and standardized formulas like 220 minus your age are unreliable for precise measurements. On the other hand, exact maximum heart rate measurements like those achieved in a doctor's office or exercise physiology stress test can be expensive to determine. But here's the issue: Ultimately, there's not much you can do based on maximum heart rates. Whatever your maximum heart rate happens to be, training won't change it one bit.

The Ultimate Lean Routine uses a different approach. Because all aerobic exercise in this program is done well below your maximum heart rate, we feel that maximum heart rate is an irrelevant number. The most important determinant of your fitness and aerobic capacity is your lactate threshold heart rate (LTHR). This is the basis from which your lean training zone heart rate will be set and all your workloads determined.

A Key Number:
Your Lactate Threshold Heart Rate (LTHR)

Although we want to train at the higher end of our "aerobic capacity" during these aerobic cycling and running sessions, we do not want to go into oxygen debt and be forced to stop or drastically slow down. Instead, we are looking for the **highest steady pace that we can maintain throughout the workout** for the minimum forty-five-minute working portion (and up to an hour for the maximum). Staying within the higher end of our lean training zone assures us the most effective use of our aerobic training time. It is here that we burn the most calories consistently without pooping out. The point at which we go beyond our aerobic training limits and into the anaerobic (*anaerobic* means "without oxygen") is called the "lactate threshold." The lactate threshold represents that uncomfortable point at which muscular work is so great and our ability to process oxygen so limited that lactic acid (lactate) starts accumulating in our muscles at a rate faster than we are able to "recycle" it back into a usable fuel. No amount of carbohydrate or fat can help at this point. This large accumulation of lactic acid is what causes muscles to shut down and our breathing to become labored panting or gasping. It's what forces us to stop. Fortunately, we can use both our breathing rate and our heart rate as indicators of when we are at or near this lactate threshold. Using that information, we can settle into an efficient, steady pace based on a range of working heart rates that is unique to each of us.

▼

It will never be necessary to go above your lactate threshold heart rate in any Ultimate Lean Routine workout.

Taking Your Pulse

Almost all top endurance athletes use heart rate monitors to fine-tune their training. You should, too. Some bikes actually have a heart rate monitor built in, making accurate measuring of your heart rate a breeze. Self-contained heart rate monitors are also easy to find in the $100-$150 range at most sporting goods or specialty running and cycling shops. Finally, there's always the tried (although a little less than true) "finger on the wrist or neck" method, in which you take a finger pulse count at your wrist or neck for fifteen seconds and multiply by 4 to get beats per minute (or BPMs). Whichever method you choose, you should be prepared to keep track of your heart rate throughout the aerobic portions of *The Ultimate Lean Routine*.

The Talk Test

The "talk test" is the easiest means of finding your lactate threshold heart rate. This test should be performed on the exercise bike a day or two before you begin the first of the twenty-four cycling workouts in this program, as a means of setting the standards for the remainder of these workouts. It helps greatly to have a friend or partner accompany you during the talk test, to write down data, and to carry on a continuous conversation with you while you are testing.

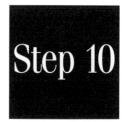

Step 10

Establish your lactate threshold heart rate using the "talk test."

The talk test involves first warming up for five to seven minutes and then gradually increasing the bike's resistance every two minutes while carrying on a continuous conversation with your partner or with someone standing or riding next to you. As long as you are able to easily carry on this conversation, you are still training aerobically. That is, you are able to take in and process oxygen for the efficient burning of fats and carbohydrates without accumulating a lot of lactic acid. When you methodically increase the resistance (by simply plugging in the next-higher level of difficulty every two minutes), you will eventually reach a point where you will have trouble continuing the conversation with your friend. You will recognize this "point of unstable ventilation" as the scientists call it, because you will probably be gasping (panting) a little and having to speak in short bursts or even just a word at a time. This point will be at or near your lactate threshold. When you reach this point, measure your heart rate (using either a heart rate monitor or the finger-on-the-pulse method) and note the resistance level on the bike. Then slow down and take a few minutes to spin easily at little or no resistance. After your heart rate and breathing have recovered somewhat (back to about where they were at the end of the first warm-up phase), repeat the entire procedure, again spending two minutes at each resistance level until you can no longer continue a conversation. Again, note your heart rate and the resistance level which caused the "unstable ventilation." Cool down a bit and repeat the procedure one more time. Now take the three heart rate numbers you attained at the point of unstable ventilation and find the average (add them up and divide by three). This number will represent your lactate threshold heart rate (LTHR).

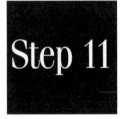

Step 11

Figure your lean training zone heart rate range.

Now, clearly, most of us wouldn't be able to maintain our lactate threshold heart rate for very long, let alone for all forty-five minutes to an hour of the workout, so we need to find a way to establish an effective training heart rate that keeps us at the high end of our aerobic zone, but still below this lactate threshold.

Figuring Your Lean Training Zone HR

Almost by definition, the lactate threshold heart rate number you just arrived at will represent the high end of your lean training zone, the highest level you can maintain and still be "aerobic." After all, we know that when you go above that heart rate number and cross the lactate threshold, you will no longer be aerobic—you'll be anaerobic, and you won't last much longer at that rate.

Now, to determine the low end of your target training range, simply multiply your high-end number by 90% (or .90).

High end of lean training zone =
lactate threshold heart rate (LTHR) _____ BPM (*high*)

Low end of lean training zone = LTHR x .90

LTHR _____ x .90 = _____ BPM (*low*)

Now you know the optimum range of heart rates within which you will want to work on the stationary bike, after your brief warm-up period. Keep in mind that during the twelve-week program you will never need to exceed your lactate threshold heart rate in any of your aerobic workouts. However, note that throughout the duration of this program your fitness will constantly improve. If you find yourself able to do the workouts consistently at or near the high end of your lean training zone, it may be necessary to retest for a new lactate threshold heart rate. Why? Because as you adapt to the workload, your heart and fat-burning fuel systems will become more efficient at the old heart rates. When it takes less effort to maintain a heart rate at or near your original LTHR, it means that your true LTHR has risen. This is a good thing; it means you've become more fit. However, in order to continue to stimulate further adaptation, you'll have to test for the new level and "reset" the lean training zone from there. It's a good idea to retest yourself six weeks into the program to see if your aerobic efficiency has improved. If there is no change in LTHR after six weeks, don't be discouraged. Just keep working within your original range.

▼

To lose fat you have to burn off more calories than you take in.

Let's go back to our example. Joe does the talk test three times and gets heart rate numbers of 164 BPM the first time, 159 BPM the second time, and 163 BPM the third time. Adding these three up and dividing by 3 (164 + 159 + 163 = 486 ÷ 3 = 162), he finds that his lactate threshold heart rate (LTHR) occurs at an average heart rate of 162 BPM. He also notes that each time he reached this lactate threshold he was riding at Level 6 on his bike. To get the lower end of this lean training zone, Joe multiplies his LTHR by .90. So, 162 x .90 = 145.8, which he'll round down to 145. Joe now knows that whenever he rides the bike, after his 5-minute warm-up, he should gradually (within another five to ten minutes) move into that 145 to 162 beats per minute range during the work session. He also knows that since Level 6 on this particular stationary bike caused him to reach his lactate threshold in his test, that he should probably be doing the bulk of his work in the first few weeks at Levels 4 and 5 (after his five minute warm-up). As he becomes more fit, the closer he can get to the 162 BPM, the better. In time he may even be able to stay at 162 for most of the workout.

Let's say that after six weeks he gets so comfortable in his lean training zone that he feels a need to move up to or beyond his old LTHR. He decides to do the talk test again. This time his three talk tests result in 166, 164 and 168, which he averages out to 166. Multiplying by .90 to arrive at a low end of 149.4 (call it 149), Joe establishes a new training range of from 149 to 166. In this new lean training zone Joe will be burning more calories, because in order to keep his heart rate within his new zone, he'll need to be riding at an even higher level of resistance on the bike. **Higher resistance equals more calories. More calories equals more fat burned.**

Measuring Work on the Bike

Progress is measured by gradually increasing the number of calories burned in each workout.

We have just spent a fair amount of time and energy establishing our lean training zone in order to be sure the work we are doing is the most effective possible. But, ultimately, the key number we are looking at in order to measure the true work done in each workout is the **total number of calories burned during the ride (including the warm-up).** This is the critical number you will record from workout to workout. You may ask, how does the number of calories burned relate to the lean training zone? Well, as long as you are within your lean training zone, the more calories you can burn, the better. And our goal over time will be to continuously increase the total calories burned in each successive workout, gradually adding more resistance (stress), so that an increased fitness adaptation occurs and more fat is burned. At first, we can increase the total calories burned from one workout to the next by adding a few more minutes to the time spent riding. But *The Ultimate Lean Routine* dictates that after we reach the magic one-hour point, we can increase calories burned by increasing the resistance level.

Suppose now that you have established your lean training zone and you begin the first cycling workout of the twenty-four cycling workouts in the twelve-week program, but are unable to complete the minimum forty-five minutes at any level. This would be an indication that you didn't yet possess the minimum level of fitness necessary to start *The Ultimate Lean Routine*. In that case, the way to begin to work up to a starting level would be to just go as long as you can comfortably go in the first workout. Then each time you do this workout, add two or three minutes to the total time riding, until you can go the full forty-five minutes at a beginning level of difficulty. After you reach forty-five minutes, you can start the twelve weeks of this program with a great deal more effectiveness.

If you do have the necessary "reasonable level of fitness" mentioned in the start of the book, you would begin your cycle workouts with the full forty-five minutes of riding at a level that was comfortable and still allowed you to maintain a heart rate within the lean training zone. Eventually you would work your way up to an hour. It is never necessary to exceed the one hour time limit to this workout—regardless of your starting condition. Instead, once you have hit the one hour time maximum, **you will continue your fitness and fat-burning progress by increasing the resistance (the workload).** You can work into this new resistance level by starting at your old pace (your previous steady level) for a few minutes after warming up, then throwing in a ten- or fifteen-minute "interval" at one level higher, and then coming back down to the original level. Notice that the new higher level of resistance correlates to a higher "calories per hour" reading, so that during the time you are at a higher level, you'll be burning more calories. Over each of the next few sessions, simply add five or ten minutes to the amount of time you spend riding at the new level until eventually the entire hour (except for your warm-up) is now at the new level. Just be sure to stay within your lean training zone heart rate. Use the same method to continue to increase the workload over the twelve weeks. This way, you can continually improve your strength and aerobic fitness on the bike while never exceeding the one hour maximum workout limit.

Regardless of your workload, you should try to maintain an ideal pedal "cadence," which will show up on most bikes as "RPMs" or revolutions per minute of between eighty and one hundred.

When your time on the bike is up, be sure to read and remember the "total calories burned" figure at the end of your ride. This is the number you will record in the "total calories burned" section of your logbook. Then cool down with an easy spin for a few minutes at Level 1 or even 0 before you "dismount."

Counting Calories = Tracking Progress

As just noted, throughout the twenty-four cycling workouts in *The Ultimate Lean Routine* you will measure your progress by gradually increasing the number of calories you burn during each successive workout. Theoretically, because you are increasing your workload each and every cycling workout (by either adding time up to an hour or increasing resistance as described earlier), you will be burning proportionately more calories each time you ride. This in turn will be a direct measure of your increase in aerobic fitness as well as your increased ability to burn off body fat. As you begin to get used to recording this critical number in your logbook at the end of your cycling workouts, you will probably find yourself habitually becoming aware of where you are calorie-wise and heart rate-wise relative to that same time during previous workouts. This awareness will enable you to treat almost every cycling workout as a small "breakthrough" as you continue to set personal "calorie burning" records over the course of twelve weeks.

▼

Although the goal is to gradually increase work output (calories), never increase the work by more than 5% from one workout to the next.

How many calories of work you add to each workout depends on your starting level of fitness and your goals. In no case should you increase the total calories by more than 5% from one workout to the next. Otherwise, the desired adaptations may not occur and you may risk overtraining and all its negative setbacks. As a rule of thumb, your progress should be almost continuous if you add anywhere from ten to twenty calories each workout. Of course, in reality you will have occasional off days when you may not feel like competing with yourself or exceeding a prior workout. On those days, just do your best to complete as much of the workout as you can and don't make yourself feel guilty about it. Under no circumstances should you attempt to "catch up" by doing twice the work next time. Just record the substandard workouts in your logbook along with all your other workouts and pick up where you left off when you feel better. The goal here is to achieve a trend towards linear progress over twelve weeks. An easy day or an extra day off here and there will not impede or diminish your progress.

Fig. 8

Joe's Calorie-Burning Progress over 24 Weeks

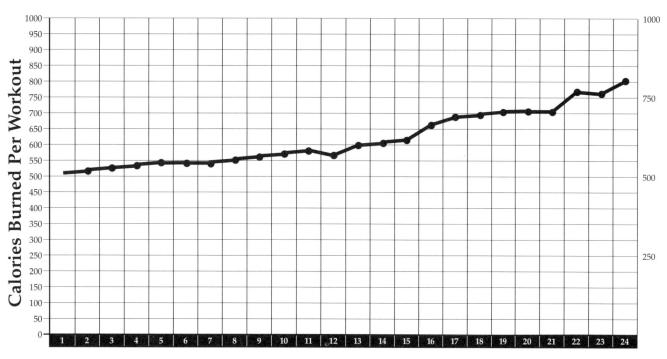

Joe started off at 525 calories in his first stationary cycling workout. By his twenty-fourth workout, he was able to burn 820 calories in sixty minutes. In twelve weeks, he increased his aerobic capacity by 56%.

Getting through the Rough Part

Although it is important to stay "tuned in" to your effort level on the bike, conscious of your cadence and your working heart rate, this doesn't mean you can't occupy your thoughts by listening to music or reading. In fact, many people actually turn their riding time into quality reading time or take the opportunity to listen to motivational tapes while completing the workout. Others just rock out to their favorite tunes. Either way, as long as you can maintain your intended resistance level, anything you are able to do without compromising the intensity of your ride is OK.

Stretches/Abdominals

After the ride session, do a few easy stretches and a few sets of abdominals (see page 63) before you hit the showers.

Stretches

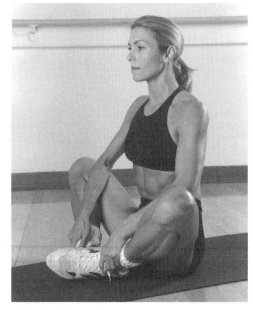

Groin Stretch

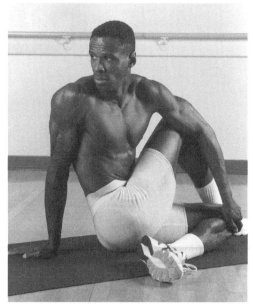

Hip Flexor Stretch

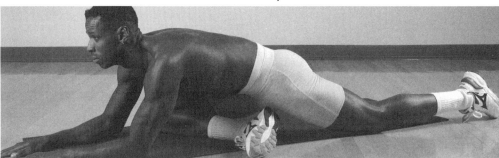

Gluteus Stretch

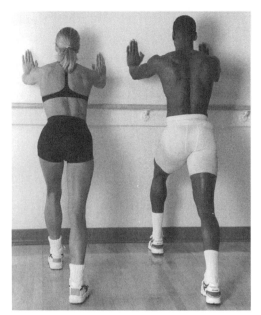

Achilles Stretch

Abdominals

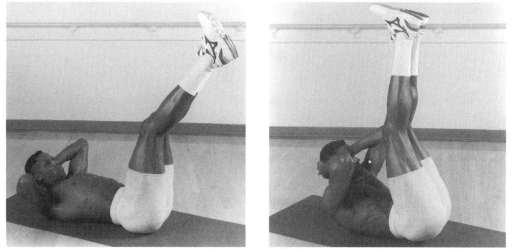

Lower Abdominal Leg Lift

Lie on your back with your hands behind your head. Bend at your hips, and point your legs upward. Using your abdominals, roll your buttocks up off the ground, while still pointing your legs upward. Ease your buttocks back to the ground to complete the repetition. Do not rock back and forth. If you are not able to lift your buttocks with your legs extended upward, try the same exercise with your legs bent.

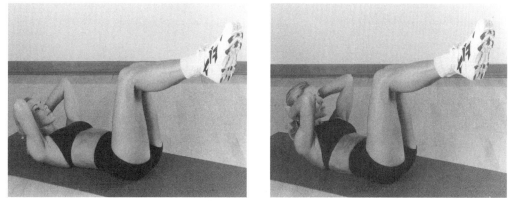

Floor Crunch

Start with the hands clasped loosely behind the neck, the back flat on the ground and the legs up in the air with a ninety-degree bend at the knee. Squeezing your stomach muscles tightly, bring your head off the ground and your chin toward your knees. Although it's not necessary to touch your elbows to your knees, get them as close as you can by squeezing—not jerking or pulling on your neck. As you get better at this, you'll increase the resistance by squeezing tighter and tighter. Come back down to the starting position and repeat for the next rep.

Days 2 and 5: Running/Walking/Stairclimbing

Day 2 and Day 5 of *The Ultimate Lean Routine* are variations of running, power walking and stairclimbing. Running is the preferred of the three because it is one of the most effective fat-burning exercises available. However, not everyone is biomechanically well designed to run. As a

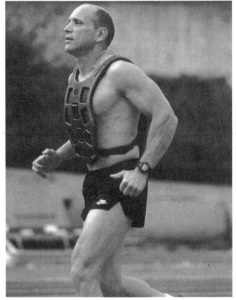

result, powerwalking and stairclimbing have been included as suitable alternatives. Whichever you choose, the goal here is once again to eventually work your way up to a minimum forty-five minutes of continuous aerobic activity and maximum of one hour. Then, having reached the maximum one hour, the goal is to increase the intensity (speed in this case) to cover as much ground as possible in that period of time. Remember, the faster we go, the more ground we cover and the more calories we burn. The more calories we burn, the more fat we lose.

Another variable that increases the number of calories burned is resistance running devices such as the Maxercise belt or Cardiovest pictured at left. The addition of evenly distributed weight on the core of your body increases the workload of walking, stairclimbing or running. Again, if running is not biomechanically suited to your body, these devices can intensify a powerwalk or stair climb to get the optimal results of a run.

▼

Running often requires that you establish a separate specific lean training zone.

The same lean training zone heart rate principle applies to this activity. Before beginning the first of the twenty-four running/walking workouts you will need to establish your lean training zone heart rates, as they apply to running or walking, using the talk test and lactate threshold. This is necessary because different aerobic exercises can be associated with different lactate thresholds, because different groups of muscles will be involved in the creation and clearing of lactic acid. Your cycling lean training zone numbers may not apply to running. As with the cycling "talk test," gradually increase your pace every few minutes while carrying on a conversation. This is best done on a treadmill, where your speed can be increased easily by just hitting a button. Note the heart rate at which "onset of unstable ventilation" occurs. Cool down a little and repeat the test two more times. Then, average the three high-end heart rates you achieved in the tests to establish your lactate threshold heart rate (LTHR) for the running workouts. That will be the high end of your lean training zone for running. Multiplying LTHR by .90 will give you the low end. You are now ready to run.

Your running and walking can be done either indoors or out. In either case, start with a warm-up consisting of walking or running at an easy pace and gradually (after about five minutes) work into your intended running or fast walking pace. If you are able to run only twenty or thirty minutes nonstop now, then at the end of the twenty or thirty minutes, simply powerwalk for the balance of forty-five minutes. If all you can do is powerwalk, that's OK for starters. Over time, from one workout of this type to the next you will add a few minutes to the run time, spending less and less time walking, until most or all of the workout is spent running or walking very fast. Once again, **all this requires that you remain within your lean training zone heart rate.** Finally, once you are able to run the full minimum forty-five minutes, you can increase the "resistance" or workload by increasing your running pace (speed), or keep the same pace but push the time out to the one-hour maximum. Obviously, if you are already able to run forty-five minutes (or one hour for advanced enthusiasts), you should work at picking up the pace gradually each week of the program to cover as much ground as possible.

Indoors, the same workout can be done on a treadmill. A combination of walking and jogging can still produce the minimum forty-five minutes of aerobic activity. The beauty of the treadmill is that you can systematically change the speeds or throw in hills whenever you feel like adding more resistance to the walk. Or you can walk ten minutes, run five minutes, walk ten, run five, etc. The possibilities are endless.

Measuring Work:
Ground Covered = Calories Consumed

Another great benefit of treadmill running is that, once again, you can keep track of total calories burned in the workout and record this number for measuring daily progress. Most treadmills provide a convenient readout at the end of the workout. For your workouts outside, the best approximation of total calories burned will be the number of miles completed (or portion of miles) times 100 calories per mile. This will hold true whether you are walking or running or doing a combination of both. For example, if you cover four and a quarter miles, you'd take 4.25 and multiply by 100 to get 425 total calories burned during the workout. That's the number you would record in your workout logbook. Although the 100 calories per mile figure is an average—you may be burning a little less or a little more per mile—using 100 will still give you an accurate **relative** accounting of your own progress.

Running is, without a doubt, one of the most effective fat loss exercises a person can do. However, some people find that steady running causes injury problems. If you can't run but still want a little more intensity than walking provides, an alternative that still involves the required forty-five minutes to an hour of continuous activity is to incorporate some stair-climbing into the routine. A fun way to do this is to rotate from stair-climber to treadmill and back, spending ten minutes on each one until an hour has been completed. In fact, even if your running is going well, it would be OK to throw in a workout like this every once in a while. Just remember, it's always important to keep track of the levels of intensity and calories so you can chart progress over time.

As in the stationary cycling days, do the stretching and abdominal exercises before you hit the showers.

Days 3 and 6: Strength Training

▼

Ninety percent of all muscle adaptation takes place in the first three sets of the first exercise for each muscle group.

Day 3 and Day 6 of *The Ultimate Lean Routine* consist of a one hour weight training session involving all major muscle groups. You might remark that lifting only twice a week and working all major body parts on the same day seem to go against conventional weight lifting wisdom. This is yet another myth! It is true that many bodybuilders believe that the only way to strength train is with a "split routine" where you might work chest and biceps one day; shoulders and triceps the second day; back, legs, and abs on the third day, and then start the rotation all over again. Keep in mind, however, that even though these bodybuilders are at the gym lifting every day, they are still working each muscle group only twice a week. The bottom line is that they are giving each muscle group the same amount of rest between anaerobic strength sessions that we are giving ourselves in this program: that is, one day "on" and two days off. The difference is, because they aren't doing the fat-burning aerobic work and otherwise wouldn't have a reason to come back to the gym on off days, they can afford the luxury of dividing their weight training routines into three days. It's also important to keep in mind that the guys and gals who benefit most from a split routine are serious weight lifters and bodybuilders, whose major goal is size. They are quite aware that up to 90% of the major muscle adaptations takes place in the first three sets of the first exercise for each body part. Each additional exercise on the same body part, whether it's a different machine or just more sets on the same machine, will yield only an incrementally smaller contribution to mass. Bodybuilders simply do as much as they can to get as big as they can; but that's not our goal in *The Ultimate Lean Routine*. We're not seeking "mass" or "bulk." We're after the biggest possible strength gains in the least amount of time, combined with a totally fit cross-trained physique. Because we are doing one major exercise three times (three "sets") for each major body part, **we are still getting up to 90% of the muscular adaptations possible.** We are able to do so in less than an hour for the whole strength routine and still have the time and energy to recover and train harder on our aerobic days.

Another common myth that many fitness buffs cling to is the notion that you should begin or end any strength training or weight lifting workout with twenty minutes of aerobic exercise. Once again, knowing what we know about the adaptation equation and the importance of adequate rest, we can begin to understand why it might not benefit us to combine anaerobic (weights) and aerobic (cycling and running) workouts on the same day. Anaerobic training sends certain chemical signals to the muscles that are different from the chemical signals produced by aerobic training. Although combining the two types of training is definitely not harmful, and in some respects may make for an occasional interesting cross-training workout, the problem is that it's simply not as effective for reaching the goals of this program. **Our intent is to combine a program of anaerobic weight lifting with aerobic endurance training synergistically to derive maximum benefits from each.** To do that we must train each system separately and allow each an adequate recovery time. If you limit your workout to one hour, as we have chosen to do, then one or both of the training elements of that particular day will also be limited when you try to lift and ride or lift and run within that hour. Moreover, if you try to go beyond the one hour to fit in both aerobic and anaerobic training, you'll lose some of the recovery benefits. Remember that because we are stressing different energy systems on different days, we want to get the most out of that specific stress and then allow the most rest.

▼

It's best not to combine aerobic and anaerobic workouts on the same day.

This brings up another issue common to any successful program. It's easy to get carried away when we see results and start thinking that "more is better," when in reality, and what often trips up otherwise well-meaning fitness enthusiasts, is that more is sometimes **worse.** Overtraining can be worse than undertraining. The one hour limit helps to ensure that you will not overtrain.

The Ten-rep Max

Your maximum strength can be figured several ways. For example, the absolute most amount of weight you can lift in one all-out repetition of a particular exercise is called a single repetition maximum. For our purposes here, the "ten-rep max" refers to the absolute most amount of weight you can possibly do—maintaining proper form, of course—for ten repetitions. Obviously, then, your ten-rep max weight will be significantly lower than your single-rep max weight on any piece of equipment. Let's say you select a weight and you are able to perform fifteen repetitions. Clearly, you have not selected your ten-rep max and you would probably need to add a little weight to the equipment to find that ten-rep max. Conversely, if the weight on any given piece of equipment you've selected allows you to perform only seven or eight repetitions before you have to stop, you would need to decrease the weight a little to establish your ten-rep max. Except for the abdominal portion of our weight training routine, all of our exercises will be based around a ten repetition maximum weight—a "ten-rep max."

▼

If you've never trained with weights, it's better during the first few sessions to use weights that are a little lighter than you might otherwise select.

It is a weight training rule of thumb that lifting a very heavy weight just a few times builds both strength and bulk. The same rule states that lifting a lighter weight many times (twenty or more repetitions) tends to build a little strength and a little more endurance. *The Ultimate Lean Routine* looks for the best of both worlds. The reason we will base our work around a ten-rep max is because we have determined that this range of repetitions is optimal for achieving our goals, which are: strength without bulk, maximum fat loss, peak muscle tone, and endurance.

For each exercise other than abs, you will need to establish your ten-rep max in the course of the first few workouts. Don't worry if your initial guesses are off by a little at first. Just proceed through the first workouts as closely as you can and then zero in on that ten-rep max by the third or fourth workout. Also, it is better to guess a little too light than a little too heavy if this is your first experience lifting weights. For purposes of measuring progress over time, **we will use as our starting record the ten-rep max for each exercise arrived at on your third weight training workout.**

One of the nice things about this program is that your ten-rep max will rise automatically over time. That is, as you become stronger, a weight that you could once do only ten times will now become "light" enough that you can do it 12 or 14 times. This is adaptation at work again. When that happens, you will simply increase the weight you are using for your ten-rep max.

Failure = Success

At times we will speak about "going to failure." What we mean by this ominous statement is that you will sometimes do as many repetitions of a particular exercise as you can until you are unable to do another single repetition unassisted. By definition, your ten-rep max is done to failure— at ten repetitions, your muscles will not allow you to do another single rep. In other words, they have "failed." The purpose of going to failure is to "convince" your muscle fibers that they need to adapt. Going back once again to the old survival model and the stress + rest = adaptation formula, we know that the body will not make an adaptation unless the stress is enough to justify tapping into the energy reserves to create that adaptation for future "survival." When we strength train (lift weights) without going to failure, we fail to provide enough of a stress to stimulate a change. When we do go to failure, we cause the muscle tissue to release chemical signals initiating those adaptations. The good news is that most of this "failure" is simply the result of a short-term lactic acid accumulation in the muscles, which will be burning pure glucose/glycogen and ATP when we lift. Resting for as little as thirty to forty-five seconds will allow most or all of the lactic acid to clear out or recycle, and we will be recovered enough to go again to failure in the next set.

Synergy

The Ultimate Lean Routine exercises should be performed in the exact order in which they are listed. The idea is to work larger muscle groups first, opposing muscle groups next, and smaller or more specific muscle groups last. As a result, what you do on the bench press will complement what you do on the rowing (pushing/pulling), and both will complement what you do on the bicep curl and so forth. So, for example, if you were to do curls as your first exercise, your forearms (and other smaller muscles involved in the exercise along with the target biceps) might get so tired

▼

A weight training stress has to be great enough to "convince" the muscle that it needs to adapt.

that when you moved to lat pulls later, your already-overworked fore-arms might give out ("fail") before your larger *latissimus dorsi* fails. If the "lat" had been one of the muscles you had been intending to take to failure in this later exercise, you wouldn't get the full benefit of taking it to failure. Doing the exercises in this order creates a synergy where the effect of the total workout is greater than just the sum of the individual exercises.

Spotting

Obviously, if you lift to failure, one of the implications is that you will not be able to complete that one last repetition. This can have dire consequences if you are lying there with a heavy weight resting across your chest or your legs. For this reason, **it is always advisable to have a "spotter" nearby who can assist you, if necessary, in lifting a weight off after you have completed a set.** Quite often a spotter can be a training partner, someone who is doing your workout with you and calling out encouragement as you struggle with the last repetitions. If you don't have a training partner, you might simply enlist the aid of someone else in the gym who is not currently performing his or her own set. As a last resort, you can always ask a gym employee or a training tech to give you a spot.

In some cases, the best equipment for a given exercise will be a cable machine or other form of "self-spotting" equipment which will allow you to do your set without a spotter. Nevertheless, it is still much more enjoyable to have someone working out with you, helping you maintain good form, and encouraging you along the way.

Form and Breathing

One of the secrets to maximizing strength through weight training is in maintaining proper form. Proper form almost always involves "perfect posture." This means your back is straight but not arched, your shoulders are back, your chest out, and knees slightly bent—definitely not locked. Your breathing should be such that you take a few easy breaths before beginning the first repetition and then **exhale during each effort. Inhale as you allow the weight to come back down.**

Timing

There are different philosophies on how quickly you should perform each repetition. One philosophy even states that you should be able to count to four while performing the contraction (positive) part of the repetition and to four again during recovery (negative). The philosophy behind *The Ultimate Lean Routine*, however, is that weight training should be specific to useful power and strength requirements. Therefore, **a two-count during each phase of effort and recovery is optimum.** That is, count "one – two" during the lift; pause slightly; and then "one – two" during the recovery. You don't have to say the count out loud, just think it. Why not the slower four count? There are very few sports where a slow contraction has any application. Most sports are explosive: You throw a ball explosively, you run at eighty to ninety RPMs, you cycle at a similarly quick pace, etc. Training must be **specific** in order to create a usable adaptation.

Equipment

The Ultimate Lean Routine describes exercises based on what we feel represent the ideal types of equipment available. However, not all this equipment is available in every gym. Therefore, we have also suggested alternative equipment for performing the same exercises. In any case, if you are in doubt as to which piece of equipment in your gym most closely approximates the exercise we are describing here, just ask a gym employee, technician, or trainer and show him/her these photos and descriptions of the exercise you are looking to perform. Not everyone has regular access to gym equipment. For that reason, we have included a series of photos and descriptions of both the "gym" workout version and an alternative "home" version of each strength exercise in which you use dumbbells. If you choose to utilize this "home" workout, you will need a full set of dumbbells (or at least a set with different weight plates and interchangeable collars) and a padded flat bench. Rest assured that significant results can still be achieved with this "home" system, provided you pay strict attention to form and you stick to the same strength training formula. And now, let's take a look at "three set strength training formula."

The Three Set Strength Training Formula

On each of the weight training exercises (except abs and back), you will use only one machine or piece of equipment per body part. That is, you will do only one exercise for each major muscle group. However, you will do that exercise three times (three sets) at varying numbers of repetitions based on the following formula:

1. **WARM-UP SET** (first set of any exercise): Using about 80% of your ten-rep max weight, do as many reps as you can to warm up, stopping a few reps short of failure. This may be thirteen or fifteen or even twenty. It doesn't matter as long as it's just before the point of failure.

   Recovery: Rest forty-five to sixty seconds

   While you rest, do some easy stretches of the muscle group you have just worked.

2. **WORK SET** (second set of any exercise): Your next set is your ten-rep max set, obviously done to failure. This is where you test yourself and your ten-rep limits. If, for some reason, you can do more than ten, do so but then move on to a higher weight in the next workout of this type. On the other hand, the first time at any new weight might allow you only nine or even eight repetitions. That's OK. Have a spotter help you through the last one or two. This counts as "good" as long as you go to failure. If that's the case, try for ten unassisted reps in the work set of this weight the next time you are scheduled for a weight session.

   Recovery: Rest forty-five to sixty seconds.

   Do more easy stretches.

3. **BLAST SET** (third set of any exercise): Now do as many as you can once again using about 80% of your ten-rep max (and to failure again). Because you will be tired from the first two sets, you may be able to do only ten. Depending on your physiology and your recovery rate, however, you might still be able to do many more than ten. The exact number you complete doesn't matter as long as you go to failure.

   Recovery: Rest forty-five to sixty seconds while moving to the next piece of equipment.

   Record each weight and the number of reps performed in your logbook and move on to the next exercise.

Now, let's lift some weights!

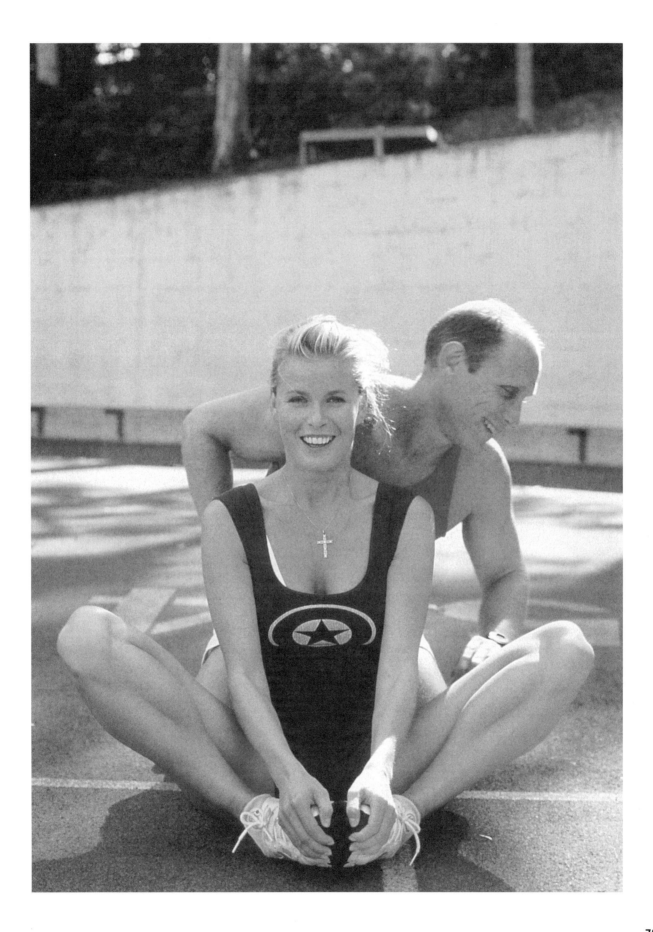

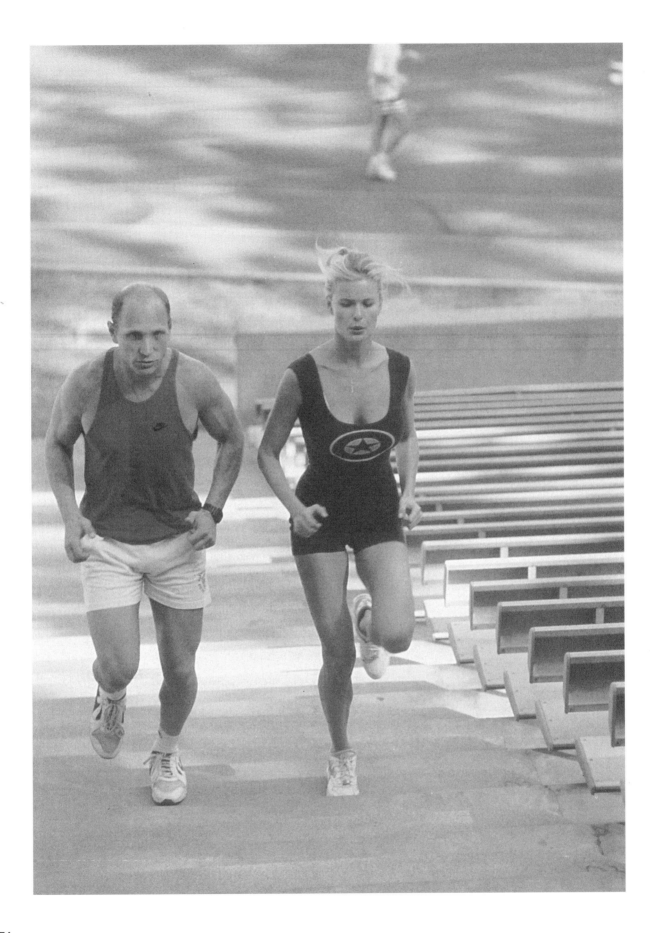

LEG LIFT

Area of concentration: ABDOMINALS

1a

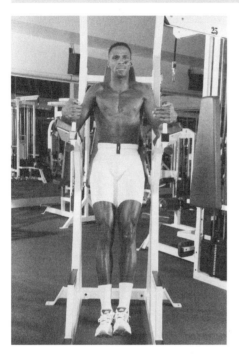

This will be a "minicircuit" consisting of:

a. Twenty-five leg lifts (an upright chair is best, but you can also do these hanging from a chin-up bar)

b. Ten back extensions (modified Roman chair is best)

c. Twenty-five floor crunches (knees at ninety degrees, shins parallel to the ground)

Go quickly from a to b to c, rest briefly, repeat the series, rest again, and repeat the series once more for a total of three circuits.

Exercise 1a: Leg Lift

Start from a straight hanging position. Don't let your body slump down between your shoulders; support yourself in the "proud" position above your shoulders, facing straight ahead. Using the lower abs, bring the knees up even with the hands or higher, and then lower them slowly (count one–two up, one–two down). Keep your lower back against the back support at all times. Don't let your feet swing back behind you as you begin the second rep. Let the feet stop directly underneath you for a brief second and then raise them again for the next rep. As you get stronger, you can increase the "resistance" by not bending your legs quite as much as you raise them.

Gym Version

Strength Training Exercises

1b

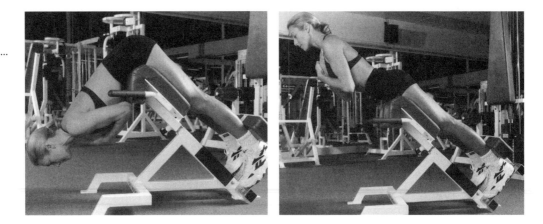

BACK EXTENSION

Area of Concentration: LOWER BACK

Exercise 1b: Back Extension

Adjust the machine so that the pads of the hip rest support your pelvis but still allow you to hang completely over the front of the machine.

With your feet firmly planted at the base, allow your torso to hang over the front of the machine and relax. Your hands can be crossed on your chest or behind your neck. Try to "round" your spine as much as possible before beginning the extension.

Now, slowly raise your upper body (while you contract your buttocks together) until it is in line with your lower half. After pausing briefly at the top, lower yourself slowly to the relaxed hanging position and repeat for the next rep.

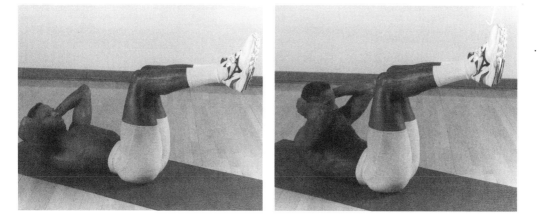

FLOOR CRUNCH

Area of concentration: ABDOMINALS

Exercise 1c: Floor Crunch

Start with the hands clasped loosely behind the neck, the back flat on the ground, and the legs up in the air with a ninety-degree bend at the knee.

Squeezing your stomach muscles tightly, bring your head off the ground and your chin toward your knees.

Although it's not necessary to touch your elbows to your knees, get them as close as you can by squeezing—not jerking or pulling on your neck. As you get better at this, you'll increase the resistance by squeezing tighter and tighter.

Come back down to the starting position and repeat for the next rep.

Gym Version
Strength Training Exercises

STRENGTH TRAINING FORMULA

After completing these abdominal and lower back exercises, follow the strength training formula for each of the next nine exercises. Remember to watch your breathing and form.

Remember the **strength training formula**:

Warm-up the first set (**warm-up set**) with 80% of ten-rep max weight to just a few reps short of failure.

Rest 45-60 seconds and stretch a little between sets.

The next set is your ten-rep max set (**work set**). Remember, this is the most amount of weight you can do and still keep form for 10 repetitions (if you can only do 6, it's too much weight; if you can do 14 or 15, it's not enough.)

Rest 45 seconds to a minute.

The last set (**blast set**) is again 80% of your ten-rep max weight done to failure (eight is OK if that is truly all you can do; 15 or 20 would be just as OK if you can do that many).

Record the weight and the number of reps for each set in your logbook and move on to the next exercise.

BENCH PRESS

Areas of Concentration: CHEST AND SHOULDERS

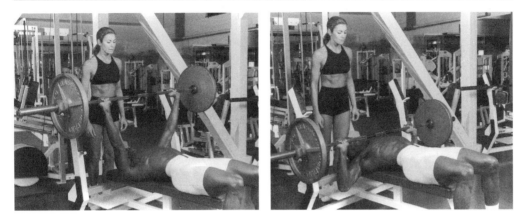

Free weights or machines work as well as the bar.

Exercise 2: Bench Press

Grab the bar with an overhand grip, slightly wider than shoulder width.

Push the barbell off the rack so that it is directly above your chest.

Slowly lower the weight to the middle of your chest and then slowly press it back to the starting position. Remember the count: "One–two down, one–two up."

Be sure to keep a flat back—no arching allowed.

Breathe in while your arms are extended at the top of the movement or while you are lowering the weight and always exhale while pressing it up again.

Gym Version

Strength Training Exercises

3

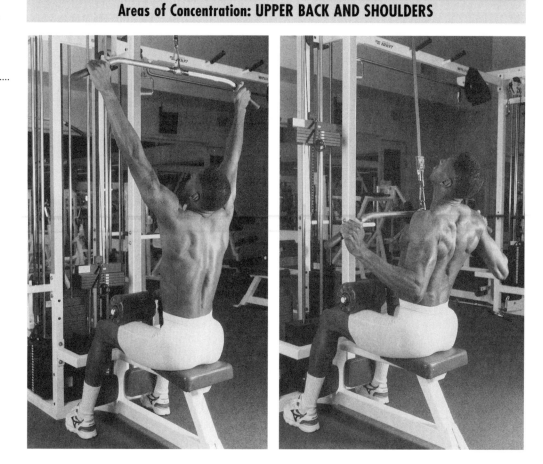

LAT PULL

Areas of Concentration: UPPER BACK AND SHOULDERS

A cable machine is best.

Exercise 3: Lat Pull

Grab the bar with a wide overhand grip.

Make sure the tops of your thighs are stabilized underneath the padded braces.

Keeping your head up and your chest out, pull the bar down to the top of your chest, leaning back slightly.

Slowly return the bar to the starting position.

PEC FLY

Area of Concentration: CHEST (PECS)

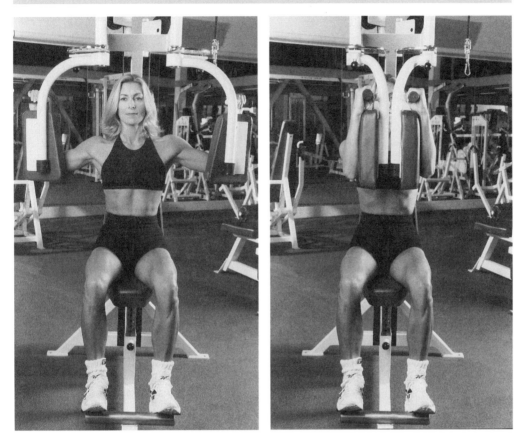

Gym Version
Strength Training Exercises

4

A "pec deck" type machine is best.

Exercise 4: Pec Fly

Sit on the bench and place your forearms on the pads so that your forearms and upper arms form a ninety-degree angle.

Keep your head against the back of the backrest (don't hunch forward).

Leading with your elbows, slowly squeeze your arms together until the two pads touch in front of you.

Let the pads return to the starting position and repeat for the next rep.

Gym Version

Strength Training Exercises

5

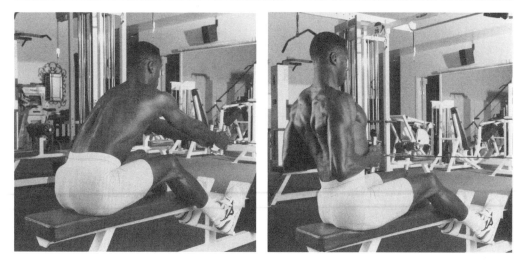

SEATED PULLEY ROW

Area of Concentration: MIDDLE BACK

Rowing: Seated cable pulls are preferred.

Exercise 5: Seated Pulley Row

Attach a double-hand grip to the cable.

Grasp with both palms facing each other. Slide back on the seat maintaining a slight bend in the knees. Maintain this position throughout the movement.

Pull handle toward your belly button. Keep your elbows tucked against your sides and your chest out. At the peak of the movement, your shoulders should be rolled back, your chest out, and a very slight arch in the back.

Key points to remember:
1. Slightly bent knees
2. Chest out and shoulders back
3. Back 90°-95°

LATERAL RAISE

Area of Concentration: SHOULDERS (DELTOIDS)

Free weight (dumbbell) lateral raises are best. Lateral raise machine is a good second choice.

Exercise 6: Lateral Raise

Hold a dumbbell in each hand, with your palms facing inward.

Your feet should be planted firmly about shoulder width apart but with a slight bend in the knees.

Again, the chin is up and the chest is out, with a slight arch in the back as you bend forward twenty or thirty degrees at the waist.

Bending your elbows slightly, raise the dumbbells to your side to just above shoulder height, "leading" with the elbows.

Pause at the top and then lower them. Repeat for the next rep.

Gym Version
Strength Training Exercises

7

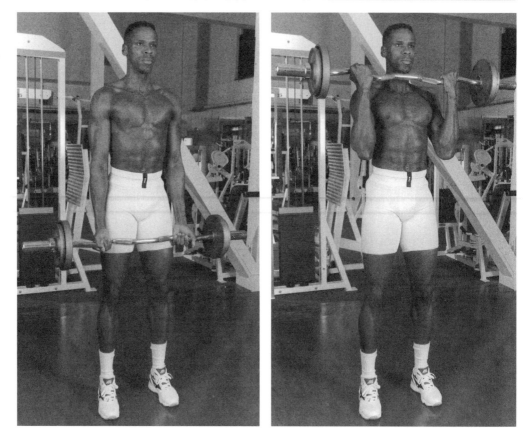

BICEP CURL
Area of Concentration: FRONT OF ARMS (BICEPS)

A free weight curling bar is best choice; a free weight straight bar is OK, as are dumbbell curls.

Exercise 7: Bicep Curl

Take a shoulder-width grip using the special curling bar.

Plant your feet firmly the ground with one foot slightly in front of the other and both knees slightly bent.

Keep your chin up and your chest out. Keep your elbows in close to your side and don't let them swing back behind you to "cheat" on the start of the lift. Also, don't lean forward to begin the lift.

Maintain a straight profile and just isolate the biceps as you curl the weight up with a "one–two" count.

Pause briefly and then lower to the starting position.

TRICEP EXTENSION

Area of Concentration: BACK OF ARMS (TRICEPS)

Standing cable "press downs" are best. Seated triceps overhead extension machine is OK

Exercise 8: Tricep Extension

Stand close to the overhead pulley cable and grasp the bar with an overhand grip.

Your feet should be planted firmly, one just ahead of the other, knees slightly bent. Your hands should be six to eight inches apart. The key is to keep your elbows in close to the side of your body.

Slowly press the bar down as far as possible (until your arms are straight).

Slowly ("one–two") return the bar to the middle of your chest, not allowing your elbows to rise from your side.

Repeat for each rep.

Gym Version

Strength Training Exercises

9

QUAD EXTENSION

Area of Concentration: FRONT OF LEGS (QUADS)

A quad extension machine is best.

Exercise 9: Quad Extension

Make sure the machine is set up so that your back touches the backrest and the front of the seat supports your entire thigh to just before the knee.

Keep your chin up and your back straight.

Don't kick the weight up, but rather, slowly raise your lower legs to align them with upper thighs, squeezing the quads.

Some machines allow you to extend one leg at a time, alternating one each rep. You can either do that or both together. Just be sure to get a full extension on each repetition.

HAMSTRING CURL

Area of Concentration: BACK OF THIGHS (HAMSTRING)

The hamstring curl machine that bends a little from the waist is best.

Exercise 10: Hamstring Curl

Position yourself on your stomach with your knees slightly over the end of the pad.

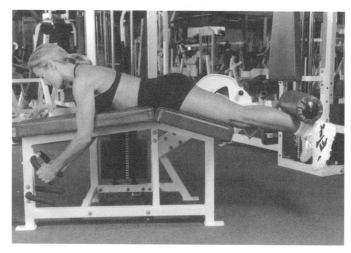

Put your heels under the roller pads and grasp the stabilizer handles along the side of the machine.

Keep your hips on the bench and slowly curl your heels toward your buttocks.

Pause and then slowly lower the weight back to the starting position.

Repeat for each rep.

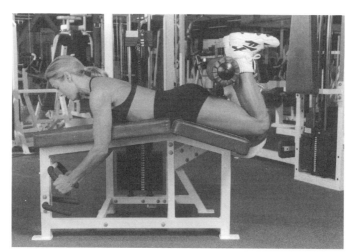

Home Version

Strength Training Exercises

1a

LEG LIFT

Area of concentration: ABDOMINALS

This will be a "minicircuit" done on a mat or carpet, consisting of:

a. Twenty-five leg lifts

b. Ten back extensions

c. Twenty-five floor crunches (knees at ninety degrees, shins parallel to the ground)

Go quickly from a to b to c, rest briefly, repeat the series, rest again, and repeat the series once more for a total of three circuits.

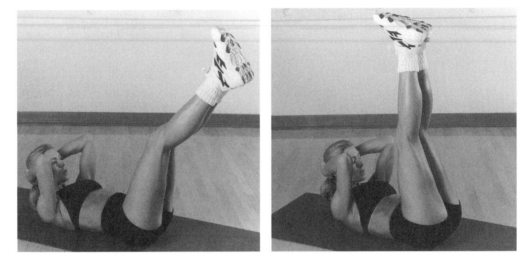

Exercise 1a: Lower Abdominal Leg Lift

Lie on your back with your hands behind your head.

Bend at your hip and point your legs upward.

Using your abdominals, roll your buttocks up off the ground while still pointing your legs upward.

Ease your buttocks back to the ground to complete the repetition. Do not rock back and forth. If you are not able to lift your buttocks with your legs extended upward, try the same exercise with your legs bent.

BACK EXTENSION

Area of Concentration: LOWER BACK

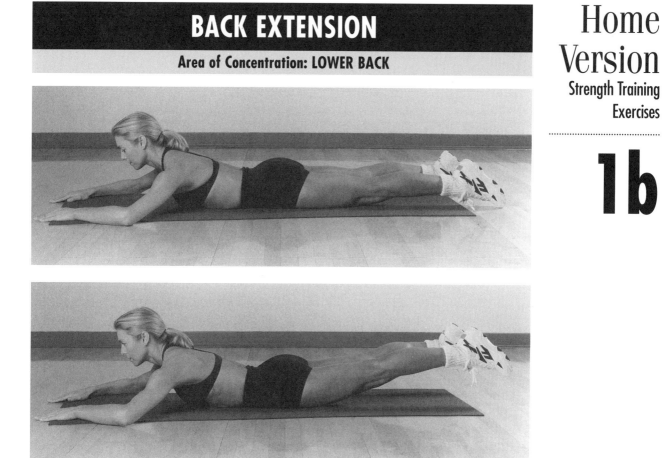

Exercise 1b: Back Extension

Roll over onto your stomach and position your arms extended or crossed in front of you.

Keeping your legs straight, lift them upward a few inches off the ground to fully flex the buttocks and lower back.

Lower the legs slowly and repeat the movement to complete your repetition.

Home Version

Strength Training Exercises

1c

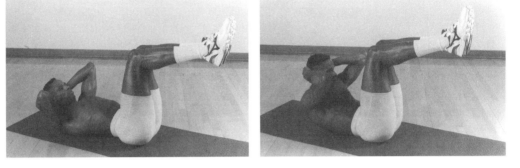

FLOOR CRUNCH

Area of concentration: ABDOMINALS

Exercise 1c: Floor Crunch

Start with the hands clasped loosely behind the neck, the back flat on the ground and the legs up in the air with a ninety-degree bend at the knee.

Squeezing your stomach muscles tightly, bring your head off the ground and your chin toward your knees.

Although it's not necessary to touch your elbows to your knees, get them as close as you can by squeezing—not jerking or pulling on your neck. As you get better at this, you'll increase the resistance by squeezing tighter and tighter.

Come back down to the starting position and repeat for the next rep.

STRENGTH TRAINING FORMULA

After completing these abdominal and lower back exercises, follow the strength training formula for each of the next nine exercises. Remember to watch your breathing and form with these "home variations."

Remember the **strength training formula**:

Warm-up the first set (**warm-up set**) with 80% of ten-rep max weight to just a few reps short of failure.

Rest 45-60 seconds and stretch a little between sets.

The next set is your ten-rep max set (**the work set**). Remember, this is the most amount of weight you can do and still keep form for 10 repetitions (if you can do only 6, it's too much weight; if you can do 14 or 15, it's not enough.)

Rest 45 seconds to a minute.

The last set (**blast set**) is again 80% of your ten-rep max weight done to failure (eight is OK if that is truly all you can do; 15 or 20 would be just as OK if you can do that many).

Record the weight and the number of reps for each set in your logbook and move on to the next exercise.

Home Version

Strength Training Exercises

2

DUMBBELL FLAT BENCH PRESS

Areas of Concentration: CHEST AND SHOULDERS

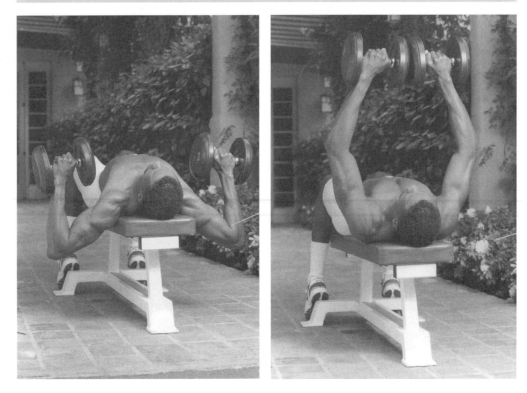

Exercise 2: Dumbbell Flat Bench Press

Lie face up on a flat bench with your feet on the ground and a dumbbell in each hand.

Bend your arms and position your hands at your armpits with your palms facing toward your legs. You should feel a slight stretch in your chest and shoulders.

Raise the dumbbells together over your chest while extending your arms and rotate your wrists to face each other.

Return to the starting position, aiming your elbows downward and back slightly.

SEATED DUMBBELL BACK LATERAL

Areas of Concentration: UPPER BACK AND SHOULDERS

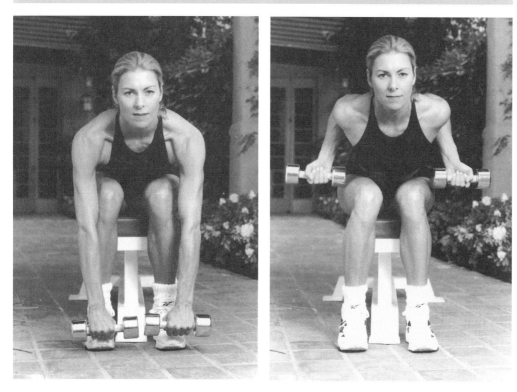

Exercise 3: Seated Dumbbell Back Lateral

Sit on the end of a flat bench with a dumbbell in each hand down at your side and your palms facing backward.

Lean forward as much as possible and allow the dumbbells to come together just above your feet.

Pull the dumbbells up as you lift your elbows upward and back along the side of your body, while squeezing your shoulder blades together.

Rotate your palms so that they face inward at the end of the movement.

Return your hands slowly to the position just above your feet.

Home Version

Strength Training Exercises

4

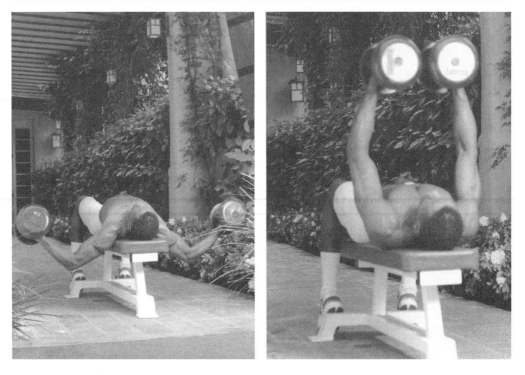

DUMBBELL FLY
Area of concentration: CHEST (PECS)

Exercise 4: Dumbbell Fly

Lie face up on a flat bench with your feet on the floor and a dumbbell in each hand.

Begin with your arms slightly bent and directly out to the side, palms up and the dumbbells in line with your chest. Allow the dumbbells to push your arms down so that you feel a slight stretch.

In an arclike motion, bring the dumbbells together over your upper chest with palms facing each other.

Return to the starting position slowly.

ONE-ARM DUMBBELL ROW

Area of Concentration: MIDDLE BACK

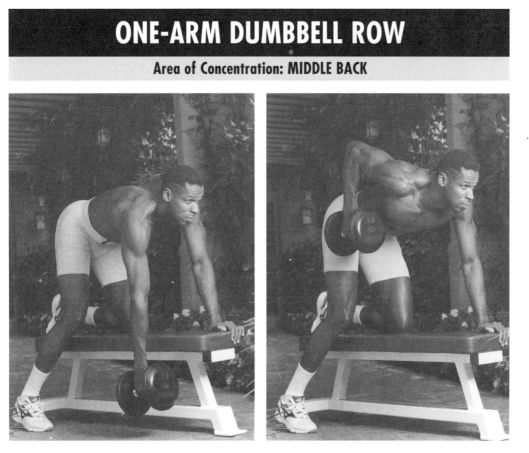

Exercise 5: One-Arm Dumbbell Row

Position the body over a flat bench with one knee on the bench and the hand of the same side on the front of the bench so your back is flat.

Your opposite foot should be securely on the floor.

Hold a dumbbell in your free hand and allow the arm to extend fully straight down with your palm facing your foot.

Pull the dumbbell upward to the hip while rotating the palm inward. Point the elbow as far upward as possible.

Return slowly to the starting position.

Repeat on right and left sides.

Home Version

Strength Training Exercises

6

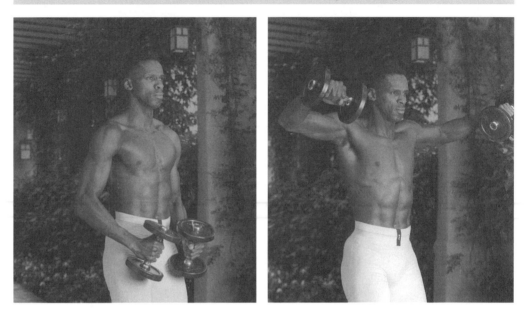

LATERAL RAISE

Area of Concentration: SHOULDERS (DELTOIDS)

Exercise 6: Lateral Raise

Hold a dumbbell in each hand, with your palms facing inward.

Your feet should be planted firmly about shoulder width apart but with a slight bend in the knees. Again, the chin is up and the chest is out, with a slight arch in the back as you bend forward twenty or thirty degrees at the waist.

Bending your elbows slightly, raise the dumbbells to your side to just above shoulder height, "leading" with the elbows.

Pause at the top and then lower them.

Repeat for the next rep.

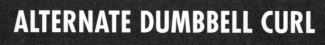

ALTERNATE DUMBBELL CURL

Area of Concentration: FRONT OF ARMS (BICEPS)

Home
Version

**Strength Training
Exercises**

7

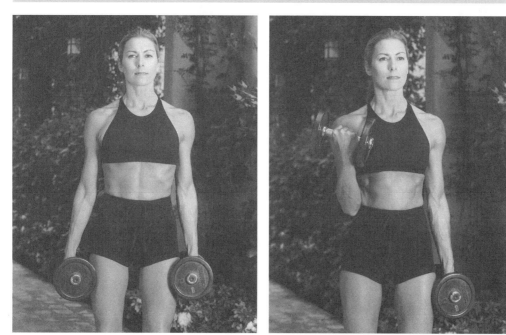

Exercise 7: Alternate Dumbbell Curl

Stand with your feet at a comfortable width and your knees slightly bent.

With your arms at your sides, hold the dumbbells so that your palms face the body.

Keep your back straight and bend one arm, raising the dumbbell to the shoulder and rotating the palm upward.

Return the arm slowly, and as you near the starting position, begin the same movement with your other arm.

Home Version

Strength Training Exercises

8

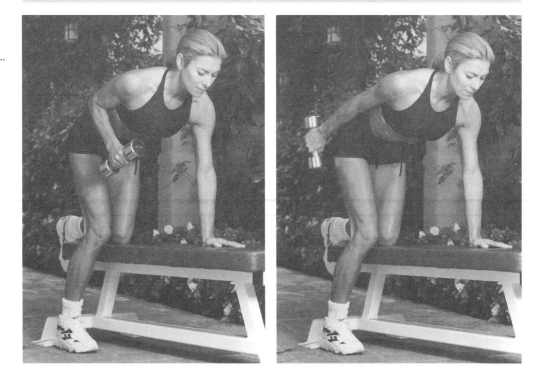

TRICEPS KICKBACK

Area of Concentration: BACK OF ARMS (TRICEPS)

Exercise 8: Triceps Kickback

Position the body over a flat bench with one knee on the bench and the hand of the same side on the front of the bench so that the back is parallel to the ground.

Your opposite foot should be securely on the floor.

Hold a dumbbell with your free hand and position your upper arm parallel to the floor and braced against the body.

Bend your arm fully with your palm facing inward, then extend the dumbbell backward using your forearm, moving only at the elbow until your arm is straight.

Return the arm to the bent position.

DUMBBELL SQUATS

Area of Concentration: FRONT OF LEGS (QUADS)

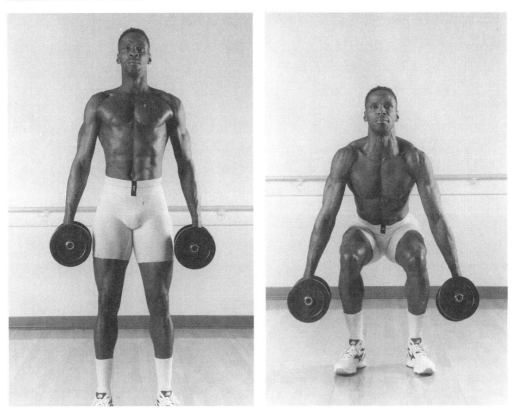

Exercise 9: Dumbbell Squats

Stand with your feet shoulder width apart and your toes pointed out slightly.

Hold a dumbbell in each hand at shoulder height or down to your sides.

With your back erect, bend both your knees simultaneously as you lower yourself until your upper thigh is parallel to the floor.

Return to the upright position without locking your knees.

**Home
Version**
Strength Training
Exercises

10

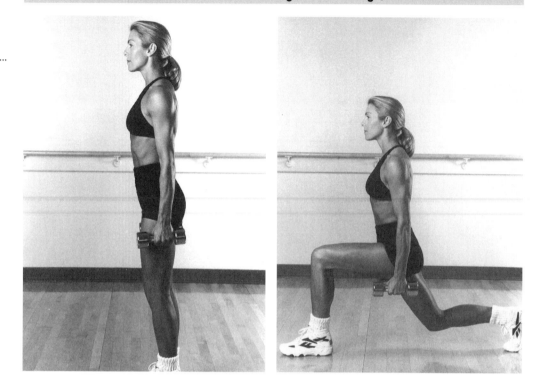

WALKING LUNGES

Areas of Concentration: Back of Thighs (Hamstrings) and buttocks

Exercise 10: Walking Lunges

Begin by holding dumbbells in each hand and standing erect.

Take a large step forward and lower your body by bending both knees. The knee on your forward leg should stay above the ankle, while the rear knee nearly touches the floor.

Return to the upright position as if you were walking forward. In other words, let the trailing leg catch up.

Press with the heel of your front leg as you come up, and squeeze the buttocks as you bring your legs together.

Repeat the movement with the opposite leg.

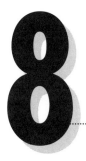

Filling in the Gaps

B y now you have learned exactly how your body responds to different types of exercise and which exercises are best suited to burning fat and building longer, leaner muscles. You have also determined your own unique dietary requirements and created an IDEAL plan for eating. You now have all the necessary information to start and successfully complete *The Ultimate Lean Routine*. However, you may still have questions regarding some of the finer points behind the principles we've discussed. This chapter is devoted to answering some of the most often asked questions in hopes of providing you further direction. If, after reading this, you find you still have concerns, chances are you will be able to address them yourself using the tools outlined in this book. Just remember: When in doubt, look to evolution and the "survival" model.

Question: If I am trying to build muscle, should I eat more protein?

Answer: Just eating more protein will not build muscle. The stimulus of resistance training, not more protein, is what promotes muscle growth. Muscle is not synonymous with protein. In fact, 70-75% of muscle is water, 15-20% protein and 5-7% other ingredients (fat, minerals, glycogen, etc.). Concentrating on eating extra protein is unnecessary for most people, and too much protein, as with excess carbs and fats, can lead to weight gain, dehydration and, if the extra protein replaces the carbohydrates in your diet, fatigue. However, some nutritionists believe that endurance athletes and strength athletes require more protein than sedentary people. As athletes increase their training intensity, they should increase total food intake, including protein intake, but only within their dietary proportion.

Question: Why are there only two leg exercises in *The Ultimate Lean Routine* strength training session?

▼

Ninety percent of all training gains can be achieved in the first 45 minutes of any workout if you know exactly what to do.

▼

Only cross-training and proper eating can create a truly fit person with low body fat, toned muscles, endurance and flexibility.

Answer: Four days a week in this program are spent doing aerobic exercises that require virtually all muscles of the legs. As a result, your overall leg strength will increase significantly just through the aerobic work. This includes calves, inner and outer thighs, gluteus (butt), quadriceps, and hamstrings. The main reasons to selectively strength-train the quads and hamstrings are to ensure a strength balance between the two and to enhance the power-generating effect of these two opposing muscle groups. When these larger muscles become stronger, we can ride and run longer and faster.

Question: I'd like to in-line skate as part of my cross-training. Is there a way to fit this in without disrupting the routine?

Answer: *The Ultimate Lean Routine* was designed to be the most effective cross-training program possible. All the exercises were chosen specifically for the biochemical adaptations they create. Any deviation from this program is certainly allowable; just be aware that the results might not be quite as impressive as if you stick directly to the program. For example, in-line skating (or Rollerblading, as it is sometimes called) is a great aerobic activity if it's done properly. One hour of skating can be a very effective fat-burning and muscle-toning routine and would be a suitable substitution for either the running or the cycling, provided you did it just two days a week as the program suggests. Triathletes might choose to substitute swimming for the weight sessions or one of the run sessions. Again, that's fine, but note that your fat-loss results may not be quite what they'd be by sticking strictly to the program. One of the purposes of this book is to help you become aware of the training possibilities and give you the tools to analyze your workout choices. There are an infinite number of cross-training possibilities available to you. If you choose to deviate from this program, just be sure you pick the ones that allow your heart rate to stay elevated for forty-five minutes to an hour. Hint: Tennis and golf are not the best choices.

Question: I figured my caloric requirements according to the plan and have been following it religiously, but I don't seem to be losing the fat as quickly as I had hoped. Can I make adjustments?

Answer: The guidelines provided for establishing your caloric needs are based on certain population averages. The number you arrived at may not be the precise number for you, but it will be close. If you are not losing fat fast enough (and understand that a pound of fat a week is a fairly substantial amount of pure fat to lose) then you might try making minor adjustments. First be absolutely certain that you are following the 30/40/30% daily eating schedule. The timing of your fuel intake is crucial to fat loss. If that's in line, be sure that you have been figuring your calories accurately. If that checks out as well, then reduce your daily intake by 200-300 calories for a week. If you notice a change in the right direction, stay at that new level. It will probably not be necessary to drop more than 300 calories from your original figure.

Question: I usually work out in the mornings. If I have the time, can I go back to the gym after work and do another workout?

Answer: This program was written for people like you, people who certainly don't lack motivation. We call them "extra credit junkies." Many of us actually feel guilty if we go home at night with any energy reserve left at all. This program was designed to get the most out of the one hour maximum workout each day so that you derive the most fitness benefits possible, achieve the necessary rest, and have time left for "a life." Two-a-day workouts are OK for some people, like professional athletes who do little or nothing else all day. But almost all non-world-class athletes will get maximum benefits from one workout a day. For us, two-a-days interfere with recovery and actually disrupt the specific chemical signals that the workouts are designed to send to the adaptation mechanisms. Give your one-hour routines 100% and then spend the rest of your day enjoying family, friends, work, or rest.

Question: I got really sore after my first few weight training sessions. Is this normal?

Answer: A little soreness is normal after any workout. It's an indication that the stress was enough to "shake up" the muscles and convince them to make an adaptation. However, anything more than mild soreness or stiffness is a sign that you went too far. When starting a weight program, it's best to do the first few sessions with lighter weights, until your body gets adjusted to the new movements and added stresses. Stretching between exercises also goes a long way towards alleviating future soreness. If, during any session, you feel sharp pain, stop immediately and go to the next exercise or end the workout.

Some people might even get a little nauseous during their first weight training sessions. Again, this is more due to the muscles not being familiar with this type of stress. Take it easy during your first few sessions and this feeling will likely not continue. Also, make sure you fuel up an hour or two before your weight training, because low blood glucose can also cause this nausea when glucose is diverted from the brain to the muscles. A small serving of a sports drink or some other drink containing glucose can help alleviate such nausea.

Question: What adjustments should I make if I get injured?

Answer: The important thing is to never continue to stress an injury. Overtraining or any acute injury to muscle, tendon, ligament, bone or any other active tissue requires rest in order to fully heal. That being said, one of the benefits of cross-training is that you can be injured and still not lose fitness. If a leg injury prevents running, you can swim and, in some cases, even ride. Have you ever heard of pool running? Many runners continue to train through serious injury by wearing a buoyancy vest and running in deep water! If a muscle pull in the arm precludes weight training for a few weeks, you can do a little more cycling until it heals. Use your imagination to put together routines that allow you to stay fit while your localized injury recovers.

Question: What if I get sick? Should I train?

Answer: Generally, colds, flu, and other related illnesses are forms of injury to your entire body. As a rule, if you feel reasonably well, and if you feel you absolutely must get to the gym, it is usually acceptable to do a brief workout at low intensity. But don't expect to see any increase in results if you do this—it probably does more for your psyche than for your body. When you're sick, taking time off to recover is always the best advice. Then, after you've recovered, you can resume your program by starting back easily for the first few days and then picking up where you left off.

Question: I'm not sure I have what it takes to stay on a program for twelve weeks. Is there any last-minute advice you can give me on how to stay focused?

Answer: *The Ultimate Lean Routine* is nothing short of a challenge. It definitely requires a degree of goal motivation. It is important to realize that in the big picture, anything is possible to some degree or another, and the level of your desire has a direct effect on the results you achieve. If losing your love handles is a number one priority for you, it can be done with focus and a commitment to achieving that result. If you have a certain image of how you would like to look, within your genetic parameters, you can arrive there one day if you stay focused and consistent. With this book, you have the technology. Now it's up to you to determine what you desire. The principles that comprise this sound and complete fitness program will work only as much as you do.

Face it, it's not easy to be in shape—it takes discipline and work. Although there is never a shortage of "quick fix" potions and formulas on the fitness market, the truth is, there is not a shortcut to a healthy, lean body. This is actually both the good and bad news. The bad news is that fat loss takes hard work. The good news is that, as with any challenge, achieving results is all the sweeter when you are aware of the effort that has gone into it. One hour of training each day and careful attention to the IDEAL eating principles are the extent of your daily commitment to a leaner you. Use this book as an opportunity to be different—to be special. It is easy to be like everyone else. It's easy to use one of the hundred excuses as to why you should not exercise today. It's easy to choose from the plethora of high-fat tasty foods and eat them late at night. Personally, I'm not interested in what's easy. I'm interested in what's hard—like your new body!

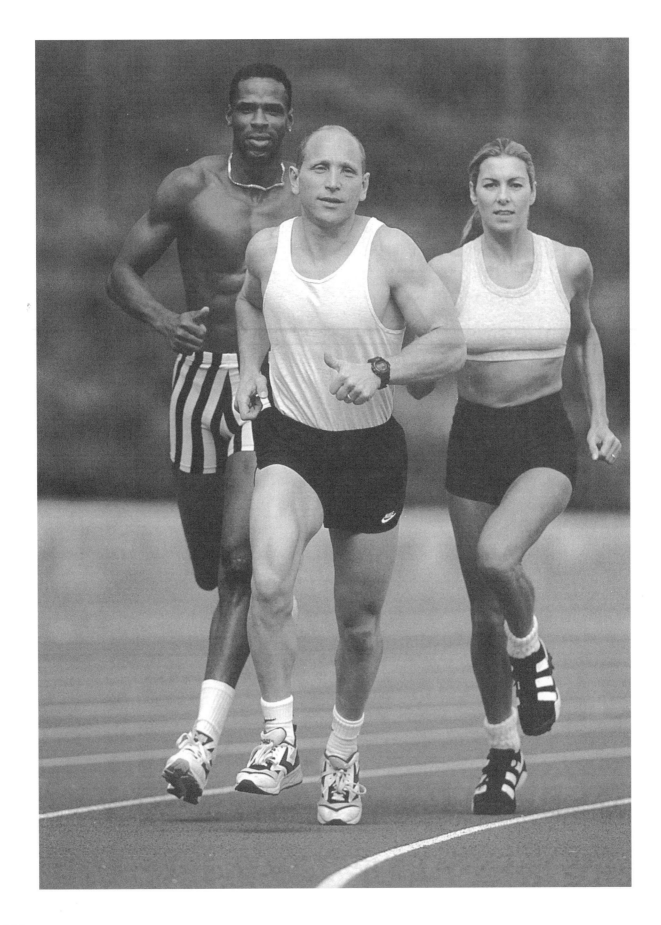

Cooking Healthy Meals

It is not always very convenient to prepare healthy, tasty meals in today's fast-paced lifestyles. However, fresh home cooking is undeniably best, especially when prepared within the following guidelines.

1. Cut back on your use of oils, butter, and margarine. Instead of sautéing in oil, use a non-stick pan or non-stick cooking spray, and/or use chicken broth as the liquid. Try to break the bread *and butter* habit. Enjoy the flavor of the bread by itself. When you can't avoid using oil, choose canola or olive oil, but use sparingly.

2. Use non-fat mayonnaise for your tuna and sandwiches, or use mustard or salsa instead.

3. Use only non-fat dairy products—non-fat milk, non-fat yogurt, non-fat cottage cheese, non-fat cream cheese. If a sauce requires cream, substitute evaporated non-fat milk with a little flour.

4. Explore the world of fresh herbs and spices to add flavor and satisfaction to your cooking. Vinegar is another addition that adds fat-free zest to foods.

5. Homemade soups are easy to make and fulfilling. Combine any and all vegetables, condiments, legumes and grains for a healthy and hearty meal. There is no need to use oil or cream in the preparation.

6. Egg whites are high in protein, naturally fat free, and make wonderful omelets. Avoid the yolks at all costs. Even when baking, add an extra white to compensate for the missing yolk.

7. Steam, bake in natural juices or grill your chicken and fish without oil. Freely use herbs and spices, lemon or lime to season. Steam your rices and vegetables without butter.

8. Use non-fat salad dressings, mustard, lemon juice, vinegar, or salsa to spruce up greens, steamed vegetables, rice, and baked potatoes.

9. Keep your meat portions under five ounces. Better yet, use meat as a flavoring for another dish (vegetable or grain dish), rather than as a main course.

10. Remove all skin and visible fat from chicken and meats.

Eating Out: What to Order

We all know that preparing our own food is the best way to assure that we are eating properly, but there are many occasions when we just do not have the time to shop and prepare our meals. Plus, we tend to enjoy going out to eat with family and friends. Here are a few eating tips as to what to order, whether you choose a fast food restaurant or opt for fine dining.

1. Deep fried foods are out. Steamed, baked, poached or grilled are in. Ask if a sautéed item can be cooked in broth instead of oil.

2. Try to find "the closest thing to the farm" as possible. Many fast food chains offer salads or even salad bars. Use good judgment in your choices, avoiding the creamy, oily selections. Stick to the fresh, undressed items and use non-fat dressing or diluted dressings.

3. Ask the waiter how certain food items are prepared. A pasta with chicken and asparagus sounds great, but the menu does not mention that it is prepared in a butter cream sauce. Ask for the chef to prepare your meal in a way that works for you. If you don't see anything on the menu, ask if they can grill a chicken breast, make a plate of steamed vegetables with a baked potato or rice, or toss some pasta with tomato marinara sauce.

4. Ask for all sauces to be "on the side," including your salad dressing. Hold the "special sauce." Salsa, vinegar and mustards are safe bets to use instead.

5. Choose thin-crusted pizza instead of deep dish varieties. Try a cheeseless pizza with an assortment of toppings such as mushrooms, onions, tomatoes, peppers, basil, and chicken.

6. Avoid prepared salads, like cole slaw, potato salad, or marinated salads. Opt for fresh greens and vegetables, and use dressing sparingly, or use lemon, herbs, and vinegar for flavor.

7. Avoid chicken wings. Skinless, white breast meat is preferred. Fish may appear to be the wise choice, but make sure it is grilled and not breaded, battered or fried. Avoid tartar sauces.

Sample Meals and Snacks

Whether you choose to eat at home or eat out, the following will provide a range of foods that fit into the ideal eating program. We all have different tastes, so improvise and bring your personal creativity to preparing and ordering your food. All of these meals will vary in their individual breakdown of carbohydrates, protein and fat content. Don't get hung up in the details, for they all fall within the acceptable range of the ideal eating system. Please take the time to adjust the portions to your caloric amounts, and eat what is appropriate for your body. The big picture here is to create an eating lifestyle rather than dictate a specific diet. It will take a little bit of time to find the healthy meals that not only taste great, but also make you feel great. Once you find them, you can eat them for life.

Sample Healthy Breakfasts *30% of Daily Calories*

It is best to start your day with some carbohydrate/protein substance. Fruit is always good, but complement it with some complex carbohydrates or a light protein to avoid the late morning energy drop.

1. Hot oatmeal or high fiber cold cereal with fruit and non-fat milk. Low calorie sweetener or a little sugar is acceptable.
2. Egg white omelet in a non-stick pan, with any combination of spinach, mushrooms, tomatoes, salsa, herbs, with dry toast or bagel.
3. Fruit bowl (melons, bananas, kiwis) topped with non-fat yogurt, or low-fat cottage cheese, with a non-fat muffin.
4. Whole wheat or oatmeal pancakes with fruit syrup, non-fat yogurt.
5. Low-fat granola with non-fat yogurt and fruit.
6. Bagel with low-fat cream cheese, tomatoes, or toasted with fruit spread.
7. Fresh fruit smoothie with low-fat cinnamon roll, or bagel.
8. Beverages can include coffee, tea, fresh fruit juice, mixed vegetable juices, non-fat milk, mineral water.

Sample Healthy Lunches *40% of Daily Calories*

Your mid-day meal is the cornerstone of your daily eating. It is optimal to consume the most calories and nutrients during the most active part of the day, (between 11 and 3 p.m.) when your metabolism is at its highest.

1. Tuna fish sandwich, made with non-fat mayonnaise on seven-grain bread, vegetarian pea soup, and a piece of fruit.

2. Grilled chicken breast or turkey burger on a whole wheat roll with mustard, lettuce and tomato. Vegetable soup or green salad.
3. Salad niçoise (dilute dressing with lemon), lentil soup, bread.
4. Grilled vegetarian burger on a multi-grain bun. Vegetable puree soup.
5. Turkey sandwich on whole wheat bread, with low-fat cheese, grated carrots, mustard, lettuce and tomato. Fruit salad with yogurt.
6. Steamed vegetables and brown rice, with salsa, low-sodium soy sauce or lemon. Whole grain toast with sliced tomatoes.
7. Vegetable salad with grilled tuna or chicken in lite vinaigrette dressing. Pita bread and a piece of fruit.
8. Sushi (avoid avocado, tempura, and mayonnaise sauce). Miso soup, cucumber salad, and fresh melon.
9. Grilled or baked fish with grilled vegetables and steamed rice, Japanese ponzu sauce or low-sodium soy sauce on the side.
10. Pasta with marinara sauce, steamed broccoli or green salad, and crusty Italian bread.
11. Cheeseless pizza with grilled chicken, onions and zucchini. Green salad.
12. Vegetarian burrito with low-fat cheese, rice and non-fat refried beans, salsa and shredded lettuce. Or chicken or fish tacos with low-fat sour cream. Green salad with fresh salsa.
13. Baked potato with steamed vegetables and salsa, lentil soup.
14. Minestrone, tomato/cucumber salad, and focaccia.
15. Japanese udon or soba noodles in broth, with vegetables and tofu. Green salad with miso dressing.
16. Bagel with smoked salmon and tomato, low-fat cream cheese, fresh fruit salad.
17. Fruit plate with low-fat cottage cheese. Whole wheat rolls.
18. Drink plenty of water throughout the day. Tea, coffee, fruit juices, vegetable juices, and non-fat milk are fine.

Sample Healthy Dinners *30% of Daily Calories*

After a long day, it is best to wind your system down with a lighter meal. Again, if you feel you need a large quantity of food, eat greater portions of vegetables or salad. I try to stick to either strictly a protein meal or a carbohydrate meal, to keep the digestive system efficient and swift.

1. Grilled or baked fish or shrimp with steamed vegetables.
2. Chicken stirfry with vegetables in ginger broth, or vegetable tofu rice stirfry.

3. Baked potato with mushrooms sautéed in broth and soy sauce, served with steamed vegetables.
4. Green salad with grilled chicken or turkey strips, low-fat cheese and garbanzo beans in non-fat dressing.
5. Green peppers stuffed with ground lean turkey and rice.
7. Chicken marinara with vegetables and salad.
8. Vegetarian chili with whole wheat rolls.
9. Legume/vegetable soup and salad.
10. Instead of dessert, choose fresh fruit to satisfy your craving.

Sample Healthy Snacks

Portion control is critical to healthful snacking. Avoid eating directly from bulk packaging. There are many snack products available now that are "fat free," "baked, not fried" to enjoy, but just be conscious of the calorie content per serving size.

1. Protein shake, made with fruit juice and/or a banana, to boost energy in the late morning or afternoon.
2. Air-popped popcorn, with or without seasoning (i.e. Braggs Liquid Aminos, salt free condiments, etc.).
3. Rice cakes, available in multiple flavors. Try sliced tomatoes, low-fat cottage cheese, cucumbers on top with a sprinkle of seasoning, or slice bananas.
4. Baked tortilla chips with salsa.
5. Seasonal fresh fruit, i.e., apples, pears, oranges, bananas, grapes, strawberries, melons, etc.
6. Fresh vegetable and/or fruit juice, i.e., carrot, celery, beet, apple, orange, melon, mango, etc.
7. Non-fat yogurt or non-fat milk.
8. Fat-free pretzels (low sodium preferable).
9. Whole grain bread, rolls or bagels, toasted or plain.
10. Cup of soup, low or non-fat without cream base, i.e., pea, lentil, chicken rice, vegetable, black bean, etc.
11. Carrots, celery, jicama, snap peas, cherry tomatoes. You can munch as much as you need from the garden.
12. Corn on the cob. A perfect energy booster and delicious cold, right off the cob.
13. High-fiber, low-sugar cereal with non-fat milk and low-calorie sweetener.

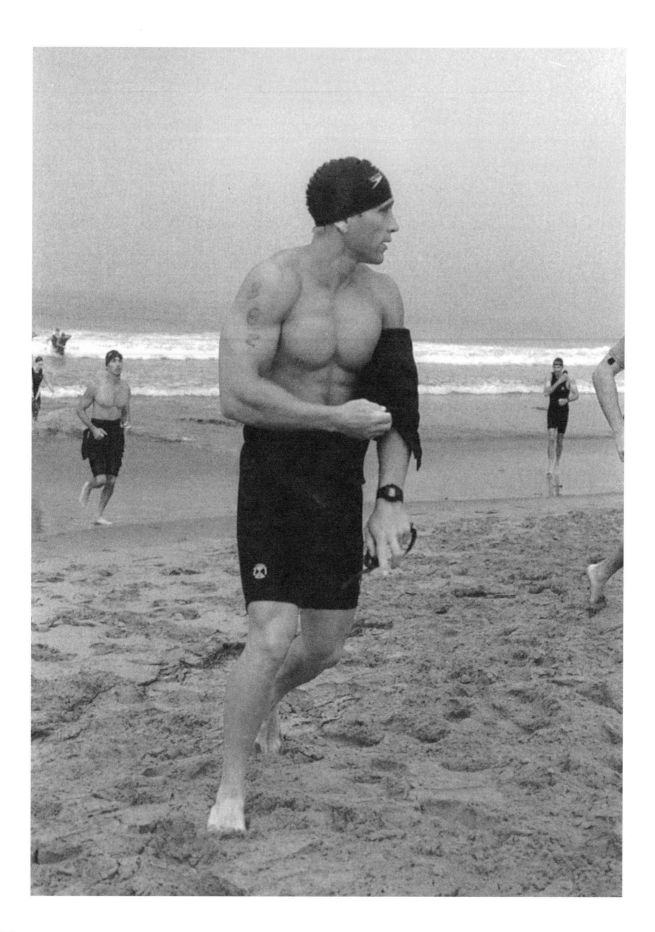

Logbook Section

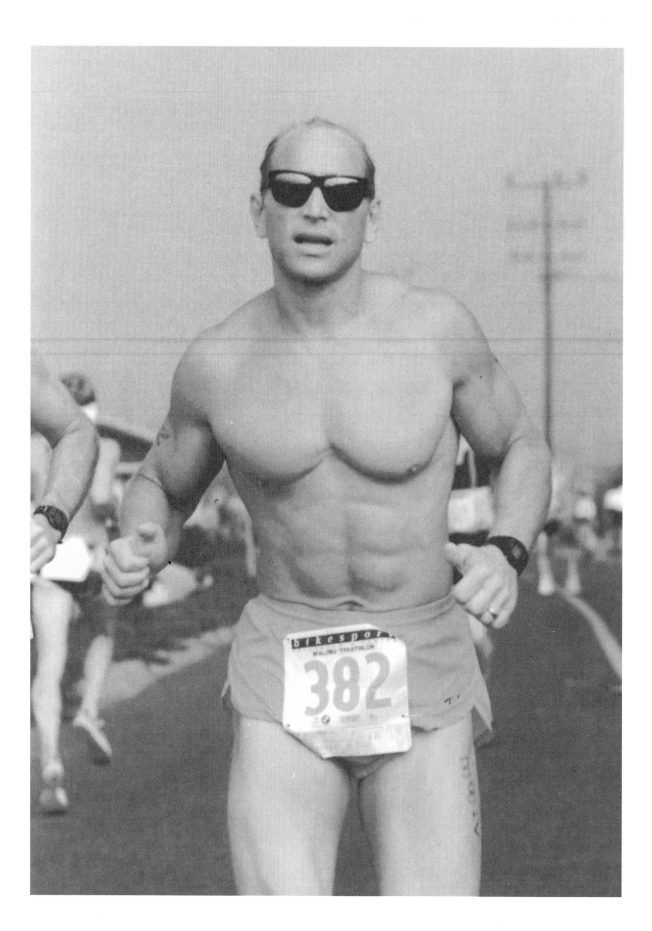

How to Use This Logbook

BEFORE YOU START TO USE THIS LOGBOOK, it is important that you read and understand all the information in *The Ultimate Lean Routine* manual.

Next, take the time to carefully calculate all your personal training information as outlined in the starting worksheets on pages 116-120. Much of your success will depend on your being able to design *The Ultimate Lean Routine* program that is perfect for you. In order to do this, you must know your weight, body fat, lean body mass, your lactate threshold heart rate and your ten-rep max. From there you can figure your caloric requirements, your optimum breakdown of carbohydrates, protein, and fats, and your starting levels for cycling and running. The worksheets will talk you through this. If you have further questions, refer back to the manual.

Now go ahead and start your twelve week *Ultimate Lean Routine* program. Take this logbook with you every time you train. Be sure to fill it in during or after each workout.

Notice that each of the workouts is numbered. There are twenty-four cycling workouts, twenty-four running workouts, and twenty-four weight training workouts in the twelve week program. Each logbook page will identify which of the twenty-four workouts you are on, as well as which week of the program you are in. You will have to fill in the date, exactly what you accomplished in each workout, and how well you ate that day. If, for some reason, you skip a day or two, start up again right where you left off. In other words, if your last workout was cycling workout Number 7, your next workout after missing any amount of time would be running workout Number 7.

At the end of the logbook, you will find a fitness evaluation section. Here you will be able to precisely quantify your loss of body fat as well as your gains in strength and aerobic fitness. Knowing what you have achieved will help you set new goals for even greater gains in the future.

Good luck.

▼

Knowing what you have achieved will help you set new goals for even greater gains in the future.

STARTING WORKSHEETS

STEP 1   Determine **weight in pounds** . . . . [   ]

STEP 2   Determine **percent body fat** . . . . [   ]

STEP 3   Determine **body fat in pounds** . . . . [   ]

Weight _____ pounds x _____% Body Fat
     = _____ pounds Body Fat

STEP 4   Determine **lean body mass** (LBM) . . . . [   ]

Weight _____ pounds – Fat Weight _____ pounds
     = Lean Body Mass (LBM) _____ pounds

STEP 5   Determine **goal body fat percentage**

If You Plan to be Diligent
_____% current body fat x .85 = _____% goal body fat.   [   ]

If You Plan to be Aggressive
_____% current body fat x .80 = _____% goal body fat.   [   ]

If You Plan to be Fanatical
_____% current body fat x .75 = _____% goal body fat.   [   ]

STEP 6   Determine **goal weight** . . . . [   ]

$$\frac{\text{Lean Body Mass} \underline{\hspace{2cm}} \text{pounds}}{1.00 - \underline{\hspace{2cm}} \text{\% body fat goal}^*} = \text{Goal weight} \underline{\hspace{2cm}} \text{pounds}$$

* *(expressed as decimal; 17% = .17, etc.)*

116

STARTING WORKSHEETS

STEP 7 Determine **daily calories** . . . . ☐

1. **MEN**: Lean Body Mass _____ pounds x 13
   = _____ Resting Metabolic Rate (RMR)
   WOMEN: Lean Body Mass _____ pounds x 12
   = _____ Resting Metabolic Rate (RMR)
2. RMR x Lifestyle Multiplier** = _____
3. Half of Total Calories Burned in Aerobic Workout = _____
4. Add **2.** + **3.** to get total daily calories. _____

**LIFESTYLE MULTIPLIER
light office work, mostly seated 1.2
housework, including shopping, errands 1.3
clerical, on feet most of the day doing light work 1.4
light construction, or lots of walking 1.5
heavy construction, warehousing, moving, etc. 1.6

STEP 8 Determine **breakdown of fat/protein/carbs** . . . . ☐

Protein (grams)
LBM _____ pounds x 1.0 = _____ grams of protein/day

Protein (calories)
_____ grams protein/day x 4 calories/gram
= _____ calories of protein/day

Fat (calories)
_____ total daily calories (*from Step 7*) x .20
= _____ calories of fat/day

Fat (grams)
_____ calories of fat/day ÷ by 9 = _____ grams of fat/day

Carbohydrate (calories)
_____ total daily calories
– (_____ calories of protein/day
+ _____ calories of fat/day)
= _____ calories of carbohydrate/day

Carbohydrate (grams)
_____ calories of carbohydrate/day ÷ by 4
= _____ grams of carbohydrate/day

STARTING WORKSHEETS

STEP 9 Determine **how much to eat when** . . . . [   ]

Waking to 10:00 a.m.: Total Daily Calories x .30
= _____ Calories Before 10:00 AM.
10:00 a.m. to 3:00 p.m.: Total Daily Calories x .40
= _____ Calories Between 10:00 A.M. & 3:00 P.M.
3:00 p.m. to Bedtime: Total Daily Calories x .30
= _____ Calories Between 3:00 P.M. & Bedtime.

BREAKFAST	SNACK	LUNCH	SNACK	DINNER
		GRAZING ALL DAY →		

Protein _____ g	Protein _____ g	Protein _____ g
Carbs _____ g	Carbs _____ g	Carbs _____ g
Fat _____ g	Fat _____ g	Fat _____ g
Calories _____	Calories _____	Calories _____
30%	**40%**	**30%**

5:00 6:00 7:00 8:00 9:00 10:00 11:00 12:00 1:00 2:00 3:00 4:00 5:00 6:00 7:00 8:00

STEP 10 Determine your **lactate threshold heart rate** . . . . [   ]

Results of talk test 1 _____ +
Results of talk test 2 _____ +
Results of talk test 3 _____ =
_____
Total of all talk tests _____

Total of all talk tests _____ ÷ 3 = _____ LTHR
(high end of lean training zone)

STARTING WORKSHEETS

STEP 11   Determine **lean training zone** for cycling & running.

High End of Lean Training Zone
= _____ Lactate Threshold Heart Rate (LTHR)

Low End of Lean Training Zone
LTHR _____ x .90
= _____ Low End of Lean Training Zone

Cycling LTZ = _____ BPMs to _____ BPMs

Running LTZ = _____ BPMs to _____ BPMs

STEP 12   Determine **ten-rep max** for strength sessions

On the third strength workout in the twenty-four workout series:

1. Abdominals/Back . . . . = _____N/A_____

2. Bench Press ten-rep max . . . . = _____

3. Lat Pulls ten-rep max . . . . = _____

4. Pec Flyes ten-rep max . . . . = _____

5. Seated Pulley Row ten-rep max . . . . = _____

6. Lateral Raises ten-rep max . . . . = _____

7. Bicep Curls ten-rep max . . . . = _____

8. Tricep Extension ten-rep max . . . . = _____

9. Quad Extensions ten-rep max . . . . = _____

10. Hamstring Curls ten-rep max . . . . = _____

STARTING WORKSHEETS

The Strength Training Formula

Abdominal/Back Minicircuit

15–25 Hanging Leg Raises
   10 Back Extensions
20–25 Floor Crunches
       Rest 45 Seconds
       Repeat Two More Times

Weight-Lifting Circuit

WARM-UP SET *(first set of any exercise)*:
Using about 80% of your ten-rep max weight, do as many reps as you can to warm up, stopping a few reps short of failure. This may be thirteen or fifteen or even twenty. It doesn't matter as long as it's just before the point of failure. Recovery: Rest forty-five to sixty seconds. Easy stretches.

WORK SET *(second set of any exercise)*:
Your next set is your ten-rep max set, obviously done to failure. This is where you test yourself and your ten-rep limits. If, for some reason you can do more than ten, do so but then move on to a higher weight in the next workout of this type. On the other hand, the first time at any new weight might allow you only nine or even eight repetitions. That's OK. Have a spotter help you through the last one or two. This counts as "good" as long as you go to failure. If that's the case, try for ten unassisted reps in the WORK SET of this weight the next time you are scheduled for a weight session. Recovery: Rest forty-five to sixty seconds. More easy stretches.

BLAST SET *(third set of any exercise)*:
Now do as many as you can once again using about 80% of your ten-rep max (and to failure again). Because you will be tired from the first two sets, you may be able to do only ten. Depending on your physiology and your recovery rate, however, you might still be able to do many more than ten. The exact number you complete doesn't matter as long as you go to failure. Recovery: Rest forty-five to sixty seconds while moving to the next piece of equipment.

THE STRENGTH TRAINING SEQUENCE

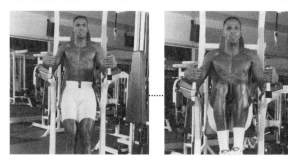

1A Hanging Leg Raise

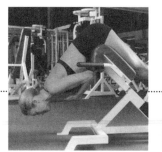

1B Back Extension

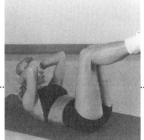

1C Floor Crunch

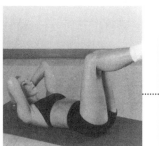

2 Bench Press

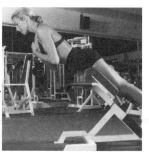

3 Lat Pull

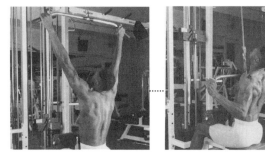

4 Pec Fly

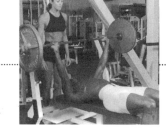

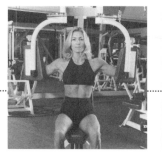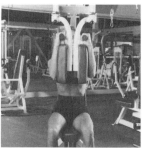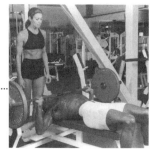

THE STRENGTH TRAINING SEQUENCE

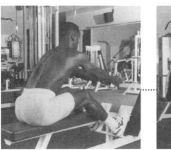 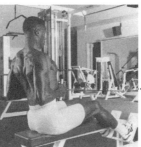

5 Seated Pulley Row

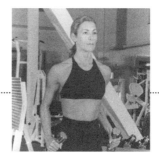 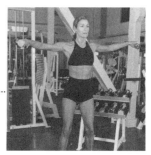

6 Lateral Raise

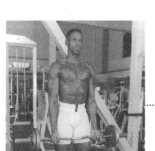 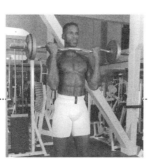

7 Bicep Curl

8 Tricep Extension

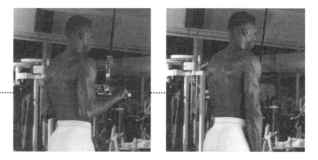

9 Quad Extension

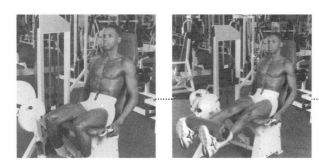

10 Hamstring Curl

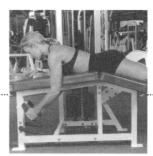

1ST **CYCLING** Workout

TODAY'S DATE:

DAY 1

WEEK

1

Today's Weight:

Average Heart Rate
During Workout:

Total Calories
Burned In
This Workout:

Total Workout
Time:
(Including Warm-Up)

Average Level
Of Intensity:

Stretched After Workout? ☐

**IDEAL
Diet
Evaluation**

	IDEAL ←			→	Off Target		
Water Intake	5	4	3	2	1		+
Fat Intake	5	4	3	2	1		+
Protein Intake	5	4	3	2	1		+
Carb Intake	5	4	3	2	1		+
30/40/30%	10	8	6	4	0		=
					TOTAL SCORE		

25–30 = excellent; 19–24 = good; 18 or less = needs work

1ST **RUN/WALK** Workout

TODAY'S DATE:

DAY 2

WEEK

1

Average Heart Rate
During Workout:

Total Calories
Burned In
This Workout:
(   ) Miles x 100)

Total Workout
Time:
(Including Warm-Up)

Average Pace

Stretched After Workout? ☐

**IDEAL
Diet
Evaluation**

	IDEAL ←			→	Off Target		
Water Intake	5	4	3	2	1		+
Fat Intake	5	4	3	2	1		+
Protein Intake	5	4	3	2	1		+
Carb Intake	5	4	3	2	1		+
30/40/30%	10	8	6	4	0		=
					TOTAL SCORE		

25–30 = excellent; 19–24 = good; 18 or less = needs work

1ST **STRENGTH** Workout

TODAY'S DATE:	

DAY 3
WEEK
1

		1st Circuit			2nd Circuit			3rd Circuit		
1	Abs/Back	a	b	c	a	b	c	a	b	c
		___/___/___			___/___/___			___/___/___		

		Warm-Up Set (80%)		Work Set (100%)		Blast Set (80%)	
		Weight	Reps	Weight	Reps	Weight	Reps
2	Bench Press						
3	Lat Pull						
4	Pec Fly						
5	Pulley Row						
6	Lateral Raise						
7	Bicep Curl						
8	Tricep Ext.						
9	Quad Ext.						
10	Hamstring Curl						

Stretched After Workout? ☐

IDEAL ⟵⟶ **Off Target**

Water Intake	5	4	3	2	1		+
Fat Intake	5	4	3	2	1		+
Protein Intake	5	4	3	2	1		+
Carb Intake	5	4	3	2	1		+
30/40/30%	10	8	6	4	0		=
				TOTAL SCORE			

IDEAL Diet Evaluation

25–30 = excellent; 19–24 = good; 18 or less = needs work

DAY 4

WEEK 1

2ᴺᴰ **CYCLING** Workout

TODAY'S DATE:

Today's Weight:

Average Heart Rate During Workout:

Total Calories Burned In This Workout:

Total Workout Time: (Including Warm-Up)

Average Level Of Intensity:

Stretched After Workout? ☐

IDEAL Diet Evaluation

	IDEAL ←———→ Off Target						
Water Intake	5	4	3	2	1		+
Fat Intake	5	4	3	2	1		+
Protein Intake	5	4	3	2	1		+
Carb Intake	5	4	3	2	1		+
30/40/30%	10	8	6	4	0		=
					TOTAL SCORE		

25–30 = excellent; 19–24 = good; 18 or less = needs work

DAY 5

WEEK 1

2ᴺᴰ **RUN/WALK** Workout

TODAY'S DATE:

Average Heart Rate During Workout:

Total Calories Burned In This Workout: (   ) Miles x 100)

Total Workout Time: (Including Warm-Up)

Average Pace

Stretched After Workout? ☐

IDEAL Diet Evaluation

	IDEAL ←———→ Off Target						
Water Intake	5	4	3	2	1		+
Fat Intake	5	4	3	2	1		+
Protein Intake	5	4	3	2	1		+
Carb Intake	5	4	3	2	1		+
30/40/30%	10	8	6	4	0		=
					TOTAL SCORE		

25–30 = excellent; 19–24 = good; 18 or less = needs work

2ND **STRENGTH** Workout

TODAY'S DATE:	

DAY 6

WEEK

1

		1st Circuit			2nd Circuit			3rd Circuit		
		a	b	c	a	b	c	a	b	c
1	Abs/Back	___	/ ___	/ ___	___	/ ___	/ ___	___	/ ___	/ ___

		Warm-Up Set (80%)		Work Set (100%)		Blast Set (80%)	
		Weight	Reps	Weight	Reps	Weight	Reps
2	Bench Press						
3	Lat Pull						
4	Pec Fly						
5	Pulley Row						
6	Lateral Raise						
7	Bicep Curl						
8	Tricep Ext.						
9	Quad Ext.						
10	Hamstring Curl						

Stretched After Workout? ☐

IDEAL ←————————————→ **Off Target**

Water Intake	5	4	3	2	1		+
Fat Intake	5	4	3	2	1		+
Protein Intake	5	4	3	2	1		+
Carb Intake	5	4	3	2	1		+
30/40/30%	10	8	6	4	0		=
				TOTAL SCORE			

IDEAL Diet Evaluation

25–30 = excellent; 19–24 = good; 18 or less = needs work

DAY 7: WEEK 1

DAY OFF!

3RD **CYCLING** Workout

DAY 1

WEEK 2

TODAY'S DATE:

Today's Weight:

Average Heart Rate During Workout:

Total Calories Burned In This Workout:

Total Workout Time: (Including Warm-Up)

Average Level Of Intensity:

Stretched After Workout? ☐

IDEAL Diet Evaluation

IDEAL ←————————→ Off Target

Water Intake	5	4	3	2	1	+
Fat Intake	5	4	3	2	1	+
Protein Intake	5	4	3	2	1	+
Carb Intake	5	4	3	2	1	+
30/40/30%	10	8	6	4	0	=
				TOTAL SCORE		

25–30 = excellent; 19–24 = good; 18 or less = needs work

3RD **RUN/WALK** Workout

DAY 2

WEEK 2

TODAY'S DATE:

Average Heart Rate During Workout:

Total Calories Burned In This Workout: (   ) Miles x 100)

Total Workout Time: (Including Warm-Up)

Average Pace

Stretched After Workout? ☐

IDEAL Diet Evaluation

IDEAL ←————————→ Off Target

Water Intake	5	4	3	2	1	+
Fat Intake	5	4	3	2	1	+
Protein Intake	5	4	3	2	1	+
Carb Intake	5	4	3	2	1	+
30/40/30%	10	8	6	4	0	=
				TOTAL SCORE		

25–30 = excellent; 19–24 = good; 18 or less = needs work

3RD **STRENGTH** Workout

DAY 3

WEEK

2

TODAY'S DATE:

		1st Circuit			2nd Circuit			3rd Circuit		
1	Abs/Back	a	b	c	a	b	c	a	b	c
		___/___/___			___/___/___			___/___/___		
		Warm-Up Set (80%)		**Work Set (100%)**		**Blast Set (80%)**	
		Weight	Reps	Weight	Reps	Weight	Reps
2	Bench Press						
3	Lat Pull						
4	Pec Fly						
5	Pulley Row						
6	Lateral Raise						
7	Bicep Curl						
8	Tricep Ext.						
9	Quad Ext.						
10	Hamstring Curl						

Stretched After Workout? ☐

IDEAL ←——————→ **Off Target**

Water Intake	5	4	3	2	1		+
Fat Intake	5	4	3	2	1		+
Protein Intake	5	4	3	2	1		+
Carb Intake	5	4	3	2	1		+
30/40/30%	10	8	6	4	0		=
				TOTAL SCORE			

IDEAL Diet Evaluation

25–30 = excellent; 19–24 = good; 18 or less = needs work

129

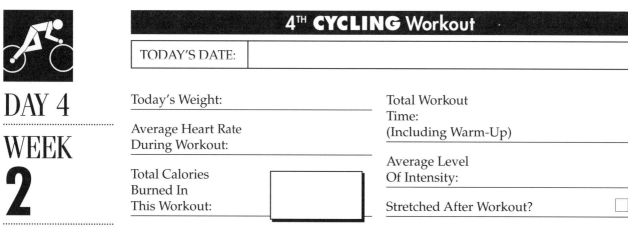

4ᵀᴴ **CYCLING** Workout

TODAY'S DATE:

DAY 4
WEEK
2

Today's Weight:

Average Heart Rate
During Workout:

Total Calories
Burned In
This Workout:

Total Workout
Time:
(Including Warm-Up)

Average Level
Of Intensity:

Stretched After Workout? ☐

**IDEAL
Diet
Evaluation**

IDEAL ←————————→ Off Target

Water Intake	5	4	3	2	1	+
Fat Intake	5	4	3	2	1	+
Protein Intake	5	4	3	2	1	+
Carb Intake	5	4	3	2	1	+
30/40/30%	10	8	6	4	0	=
				TOTAL SCORE		

25–30 = excellent; 19–24 = good; 18 or less = needs work

4ᵀᴴ **RUN/WALK** Workout

TODAY'S DATE:

DAY 5
WEEK
2

Average Heart Rate
During Workout:

Total Calories
Burned In
This Workout:
(   ) Miles x 100)

Total Workout
Time:
(Including Warm-Up)

Average Pace

Stretched After Workout? ☐

**IDEAL
Diet
Evaluation**

IDEAL ←————————→ Off Target

Water Intake	5	4	3	2	1	+
Fat Intake	5	4	3	2	1	+
Protein Intake	5	4	3	2	1	+
Carb Intake	5	4	3	2	1	+
30/40/30%	10	8	6	4	0	=
				TOTAL SCORE		

25–30 = excellent; 19–24 = good; 18 or less = needs work

4ᵀᴴ **STRENGTH** Workout

TODAY'S DATE:	

DAY 6

WEEK

2

		1st Circuit			2nd Circuit			3rd Circuit		
		a	b	c	a	b	c	a	b	c
1	Abs/Back	___	/___	/___	___	/___	/___	___	/___	/___

		Warm-Up Set (80%)		Work Set (100%)		Blast Set (80%)	
		Weight	Reps	Weight	Reps	Weight	Reps
2	Bench Press						
3	Lat Pull						
4	Pec Fly						
5	Pulley Row						
6	Lateral Raise						
7	Bicep Curl						
8	Tricep Ext.						
9	Quad Ext.						
10	Hamstring Curl						

Stretched After Workout? ☐

IDEAL ⟵————————⟶ **Off Target**

Water Intake	5	4	3	2	1		+
Fat Intake	5	4	3	2	1		+
Protein Intake	5	4	3	2	1		+
Carb Intake	5	4	3	2	1		+
30/40/30%	10	8	6	4	0		=
				TOTAL SCORE			

IDEAL Diet Evaluation

25–30 = excellent; 19–24 = good; 18 or less = needs work

DAY 7 : WEEK 2

DAY OFF!

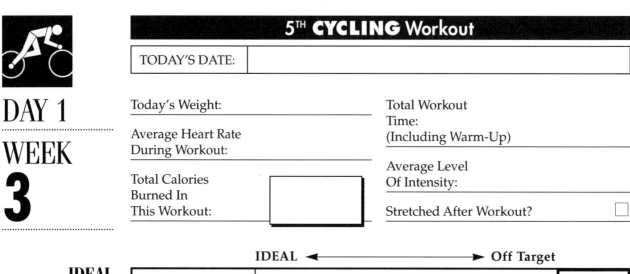

5TH **CYCLING** Workout

DAY 1

WEEK

3

TODAY'S DATE:

Today's Weight:

Average Heart Rate
During Workout:

Total Calories
Burned In
This Workout:

Total Workout
Time:
(Including Warm-Up)

Average Level
Of Intensity:

Stretched After Workout? ☐

IDEAL Diet Evaluation

	IDEAL ← → Off Target						
Water Intake	5	4	3	2	1		+
Fat Intake	5	4	3	2	1		+
Protein Intake	5	4	3	2	1		+
Carb Intake	5	4	3	2	1		+
30/40/30%	10	8	6	4	0		=
					TOTAL SCORE		

25–30 = excellent; 19–24 = good; 18 or less = needs work

5TH **RUN/WALK** Workout

DAY 2

WEEK

3

TODAY'S DATE:

Average Heart Rate
During Workout:

Total Calories
Burned In
This Workout:
(   ) Miles x 100)

Total Workout
Time:
(Including Warm-Up)

Average Pace

Stretched After Workout? ☐

IDEAL Diet Evaluation

	IDEAL ← → Off Target						
Water Intake	5	4	3	2	1		+
Fat Intake	5	4	3	2	1		+
Protein Intake	5	4	3	2	1		+
Carb Intake	5	4	3	2	1		+
30/40/30%	10	8	6	4	0		=
					TOTAL SCORE		

25–30 = excellent; 19–24 = good; 18 or less = needs work

5TH STRENGTH Workout

TODAY'S DATE:	

DAY 3

WEEK

3

		1st Circuit			2nd Circuit			3rd Circuit		
		a	b	c	a	b	c	a	b	c
1	Abs/Back	___/___/___			___/___/___			___/___/___		

		Warm-Up Set (80%)		Work Set (100%)		Blast Set (80%)	
		Weight	Reps	Weight	Reps	Weight	Reps
2	Bench Press						
3	Lat Pull						
4	Pec Fly						
5	Pulley Row						
6	Lateral Raise						
7	Bicep Curl						
8	Tricep Ext.						
9	Quad Ext.						
10	Hamstring Curl						

Stretched After Workout? ☐

	IDEAL ←				→ Off Target		
Water Intake	5	4	3	2	1		+
Fat Intake	5	4	3	2	1		+
Protein Intake	5	4	3	2	1		+
Carb Intake	5	4	3	2	1		+
30/40/30%	10	8	6	4	0		=
				TOTAL SCORE			

IDEAL Diet Evaluation

25–30 = excellent; 19–24 = good; 18 or less = needs work

6TH **CYCLING** Workout

TODAY'S DATE:

DAY 4

WEEK 3

Today's Weight:

Average Heart Rate During Workout:

Total Calories Burned In This Workout:

Total Workout Time: (Including Warm-Up)

Average Level Of Intensity:

Stretched After Workout? ☐

IDEAL Diet Evaluation

IDEAL ←——————→ Off Target

	IDEAL				Off Target		
Water Intake	5	4	3	2	1		+
Fat Intake	5	4	3	2	1		+
Protein Intake	5	4	3	2	1		+
Carb Intake	5	4	3	2	1		+
30/40/30%	10	8	6	4	0		=
					TOTAL SCORE		

25–30 = excellent; 19–24 = good; 18 or less = needs work

6TH **RUN/WALK** Workout

TODAY'S DATE:

DAY 5

WEEK 3

Average Heart Rate During Workout:

Total Calories Burned In This Workout: (   ) Miles x 100)

Total Workout Time: (Including Warm-Up)

Average Pace

Stretched After Workout? ☐

IDEAL Diet Evaluation

IDEAL ←——————→ Off Target

	IDEAL				Off Target		
Water Intake	5	4	3	2	1		+
Fat Intake	5	4	3	2	1		+
Protein Intake	5	4	3	2	1		+
Carb Intake	5	4	3	2	1		+
30/40/30%	10	8	6	4	0		=
					TOTAL SCORE		

25–30 = excellent; 19–24 = good; 18 or less = needs work

6TH **STRENGTH** Workout

TODAY'S DATE:

DAY 6

WEEK

3

		1st Circuit			2nd Circuit			3rd Circuit		
		a	b	c	a	b	c	a	b	c
1	Abs/Back	___/___/___			___/___/___			___/___/___		

		Warm-Up Set (80%)		Work Set (100%)		Blast Set (80%)	
		Weight	Reps	Weight	Reps	Weight	Reps
2	Bench Press						
3	Lat Pull						
4	Pec Fly						
5	Pulley Row						
6	Lateral Raise						
7	Bicep Curl						
8	Tricep Ext.						
9	Quad Ext.						
10	Hamstring Curl						

Stretched After Workout? ☐

IDEAL ←————————→ **Off Target**

Water Intake	5	4	3	2	1		+
Fat Intake	5	4	3	2	1		+
Protein Intake	5	4	3	2	1		+
Carb Intake	5	4	3	2	1		+
30/40/30%	10	8	6	4	0		=
				TOTAL SCORE		

IDEAL Diet Evaluation

25–30 = excellent; 19–24 = good; 18 or less = needs work

DAY 7 : WEEK 3

DAY OFF!

DAY 1
WEEK
4

7ᵀᴴ **CYCLING** Workout

TODAY'S DATE:

Today's Weight:

Average Heart Rate
During Workout:

Total Calories
Burned In
This Workout:

Total Workout
Time:
(Including Warm-Up)

Average Level
Of Intensity:

Stretched After Workout? ☐

**IDEAL
Diet
Evaluation**

IDEAL ⟷ Off Target

Water Intake	5	4	3	2	1	+
Fat Intake	5	4	3	2	1	+
Protein Intake	5	4	3	2	1	+
Carb Intake	5	4	3	2	1	+
30/40/30%	10	8	6	4	0	=
					TOTAL SCORE	

25–30 = excellent; 19–24 = good; 18 or less = needs work

DAY 2
WEEK
4

7ᵀᴴ **RUN/WALK** Workout

TODAY'S DATE:

Average Heart Rate
During Workout:

Total Calories
Burned In
This Workout:
(   ) Miles x 100)

Total Workout
Time:
(Including Warm-Up)

Average Pace

Stretched After Workout? ☐

**IDEAL
Diet
Evaluation**

IDEAL ⟷ Off Target

Water Intake	5	4	3	2	1	+
Fat Intake	5	4	3	2	1	+
Protein Intake	5	4	3	2	1	+
Carb Intake	5	4	3	2	1	+
30/40/30%	10	8	6	4	0	=
					TOTAL SCORE	

25–30 = excellent; 19–24 = good; 18 or less = needs work

7ᵀᴴ **STRENGTH** Workout

TODAY'S DATE:

DAY 3

WEEK

4

		1st Circuit			2nd Circuit			3rd Circuit		
		a	b	c	a	b	c	a	b	c
1	Abs/Back	___	/ ___	/ ___	___	/ ___	/ ___	___	/ ___	/ ___

		Warm-Up Set (80%)		Work Set (100%)		Blast Set (80%)	
		Weight	Reps	Weight	Reps	Weight	Reps
2	Bench Press						
3	Lat Pull						
4	Pec Fly						
5	Pulley Row						
6	Lateral Raise						
7	Bicep Curl						
8	Tricep Ext.						
9	Quad Ext.						
10	Hamstring Curl						

Stretched After Workout? ☐

	IDEAL ←——————→ Off Target						
Water Intake	5	4	3	2	1		+
Fat Intake	5	4	3	2	1		+
Protein Intake	5	4	3	2	1		+
Carb Intake	5	4	3	2	1		+
30/40/30%	10	8	6	4	0		=
				TOTAL SCORE			

IDEAL Diet Evaluation

25–30 = excellent; 19–24 = good; 18 or less = needs work

DAY 4

WEEK
4

8ᵀᴴ **CYCLING** Workout

TODAY'S DATE:

Today's Weight:

Average Heart Rate
During Workout:

Total Calories
Burned In
This Workout:

Total Workout
Time:
(Including Warm-Up)

Average Level
Of Intensity:

Stretched After Workout? ☐

**IDEAL
Diet
Evaluation**

	IDEAL ←——————→ Off Target						
Water Intake	5	4	3	2	1		+
Fat Intake	5	4	3	2	1		+
Protein Intake	5	4	3	2	1		+
Carb Intake	5	4	3	2	1		+
30/40/30%	10	8	6	4	0		=
					TOTAL SCORE		

25–30 = excellent; 19–24 = good; 18 or less = needs work

DAY 5

WEEK
4

8ᵀᴴ **RUN/WALK** Workout

TODAY'S DATE:

Average Heart Rate
During Workout:

Total Calories
Burned In
This Workout:
(   ) Miles x 100)

Total Workout
Time:
(Including Warm-Up)

Average Pace

Stretched After Workout? ☐

**IDEAL
Diet
Evaluation**

	IDEAL ←——————→ Off Target						
Water Intake	5	4	3	2	1		+
Fat Intake	5	4	3	2	1		+
Protein Intake	5	4	3	2	1		+
Carb Intake	5	4	3	2	1		+
30/40/30%	10	8	6	4	0		=
					TOTAL SCORE		

25–30 = excellent; 19–24 = good; 18 or less = needs work

8ᵀᴴ **STRENGTH** Workout

TODAY'S DATE:	

DAY 6

WEEK 4

		1st Circuit			2nd Circuit			3rd Circuit		
1	Abs/Back	a	b	c	a	b	c	a	b	c
		___/___/___			___/___/___			___/___/___		
		Warm-Up Set (80%)		**Work Set (100%)**		**Blast Set (80%)**	
		Weight	Reps	Weight	Reps	Weight	Reps
2	Bench Press						
3	Lat Pull						
4	Pec Fly						
5	Pulley Row						
6	Lateral Raise						
7	Bicep Curl						
8	Tricep Ext.						
9	Quad Ext.						
10	Hamstring Curl						

Stretched After Workout? ☐

	IDEAL ← → **Off Target**						
Water Intake	5	4	3	2	1		+
Fat Intake	5	4	3	2	1		+
Protein Intake	5	4	3	2	1		+
Carb Intake	5	4	3	2	1		+
30/40/30%	10	8	6	4	0		=
				TOTAL SCORE			

IDEAL Diet Evaluation

25–30 = excellent; 19–24 = good; 18 or less = needs work

DAY 7: WEEK 4

DAY OFF!

DAY 1
WEEK
5

9TH **CYCLING** Workout

TODAY'S DATE:	

Today's Weight:

Average Heart Rate During Workout:

Total Calories Burned In This Workout:

Total Workout Time: (Including Warm-Up)

Average Level Of Intensity:

Stretched After Workout? ☐

IDEAL Diet Evaluation

	IDEAL ←——————→ Off Target						
Water Intake	5	4	3	2	1		+
Fat Intake	5	4	3	2	1		+
Protein Intake	5	4	3	2	1		+
Carb Intake	5	4	3	2	1		+
30/40/30%	10	8	6	4	0		=
				TOTAL SCORE			

25–30 = excellent; 19–24 = good; 18 or less = needs work

DAY 2
WEEK
5

9TH **RUN/WALK** Workout

TODAY'S DATE:	

Average Heart Rate During Workout:

Total Calories Burned In This Workout: ( ) Miles x 100)

Total Workout Time: (Including Warm-Up)

Average Pace

Stretched After Workout? ☐

IDEAL Diet Evaluation

	IDEAL ←——————→ Off Target						
Water Intake	5	4	3	2	1		+
Fat Intake	5	4	3	2	1		+
Protein Intake	5	4	3	2	1		+
Carb Intake	5	4	3	2	1		+
30/40/30%	10	8	6	4	0		=
				TOTAL SCORE			

25–30 = excellent; 19–24 = good; 18 or less = needs work

9ᵀᴴ **STRENGTH** Workout

TODAY'S DATE:

DAY 3

WEEK 5

	1st Circuit			2nd Circuit			3rd Circuit		
1 Abs/Back	a	b	c	a	b	c	a	b	c
	___/___/___			___/___/___			___/___/___		

	Warm-Up Set (80%)		Work Set (100%)		Blast Set (80%)	
	Weight	Reps	Weight	Reps	Weight	Reps
2 Bench Press						
3 Lat Pull						
4 Pec Fly						
5 Pulley Row						
6 Lateral Raise						
7 Bicep Curl						
8 Tricep Ext.						
9 Quad Ext.						
10 Hamstring Curl						

Stretched After Workout? ☐

IDEAL ←―――――――――→ **Off Target**

Water Intake	5	4	3	2	1		+
Fat Intake	5	4	3	2	1		+
Protein Intake	5	4	3	2	1		+
Carb Intake	5	4	3	2	1		+
30/40/30%	10	8	6	4	0		=
					TOTAL SCORE		

IDEAL Diet Evaluation

25–30 = excellent; 19–24 = good; 18 or less = needs work

DAY 4
WEEK
5

10TH **CYCLING** Workout

TODAY'S DATE:

Today's Weight:

Average Heart Rate
During Workout:

Total Calories
Burned In
This Workout:

Total Workout
Time:
(Including Warm-Up)

Average Level
Of Intensity:

Stretched After Workout? ☐

**IDEAL
Diet
Evaluation**

	IDEAL ⟵――――――⟶ Off Target						
Water Intake	5	4	3	2	1		+
Fat Intake	5	4	3	2	1		+
Protein Intake	5	4	3	2	1		+
Carb Intake	5	4	3	2	1		+
30/40/30%	10	8	6	4	0		=
					TOTAL SCORE		

25–30 = excellent; 19–24 = good; 18 or less = needs work

DAY 5
WEEK
5

10TH **RUN/WALK** Workout

TODAY'S DATE:

Average Heart Rate
During Workout:

Total Calories
Burned In
This Workout:
(   ) Miles x 100)

Total Workout
Time:
(Including Warm-Up)

Average Pace

Stretched After Workout? ☐

**IDEAL
Diet
Evaluation**

	IDEAL ⟵――――――⟶ Off Target						
Water Intake	5	4	3	2	1		+
Fat Intake	5	4	3	2	1		+
Protein Intake	5	4	3	2	1		+
Carb Intake	5	4	3	2	1		+
30/40/30%	10	8	6	4	0		=
					TOTAL SCORE		

25–30 = excellent; 19–24 = good; 18 or less = needs work

10TH **STRENGTH** Workout

DAY 6

WEEK 5

TODAY'S DATE:	

		1st Circuit			2nd Circuit			3rd Circuit		
1	Abs/Back	a	b	c	a	b	c	a	b	c
		___/___/___			___/___/___			___/___/___		

		Warm-Up Set (80%)		**Work Set (100%)**		**Blast Set (80%)**	
		Weight	Reps	Weight	Reps	Weight	Reps
2	Bench Press						
3	Lat Pull						
4	Pec Fly						
5	Pulley Row						
6	Lateral Raise						
7	Bicep Curl						
8	Tricep Ext.						
9	Quad Ext.						
10	Hamstring Curl						

Stretched After Workout? ☐

IDEAL ◄—————► Off Target

Water Intake	5	4	3	2	1		+
Fat Intake	5	4	3	2	1		+
Protein Intake	5	4	3	2	1		+
Carb Intake	5	4	3	2	1		+
30/40/30%	10	8	6	4	0		=
				TOTAL SCORE			

IDEAL Diet Evaluation

25–30 = excellent; 19–24 = good; 18 or less = needs work

DAY 7 : WEEK 5

DAY OFF

11ᵀᴴ **CYCLING** Workout

DAY 1

WEEK 6

TODAY'S DATE:	

Today's Weight: _____

Average Heart Rate During Workout: _____

Total Calories Burned In This Workout:

Total Workout Time: (Including Warm-Up) _____

Average Level Of Intensity: _____

Stretched After Workout? ☐

IDEAL Diet Evaluation

	IDEAL ←				→ Off Target		
Water Intake	5	4	3	2	1		+
Fat Intake	5	4	3	2	1		+
Protein Intake	5	4	3	2	1		+
Carb Intake	5	4	3	2	1		+
30/40/30%	10	8	6	4	0		=
					TOTAL SCORE		

25–30 = excellent; 19–24 = good; 18 or less = needs work

11ᵀᴴ **RUN/WALK** Workout

DAY 2

WEEK 6

TODAY'S DATE:	

Average Heart Rate During Workout: _____

Total Calories Burned In This Workout: (_____) Miles x 100)

Total Workout Time: (Including Warm-Up) _____

Average Pace _____

Stretched After Workout? ☐

IDEAL Diet Evaluation

	IDEAL ←				→ Off Target		
Water Intake	5	4	3	2	1		+
Fat Intake	5	4	3	2	1		+
Protein Intake	5	4	3	2	1		+
Carb Intake	5	4	3	2	1		+
30/40/30%	10	8	6	4	0		=
					TOTAL SCORE		

25–30 = excellent; 19–24 = good; 18 or less = needs work

11ᵀᴴ **STRENGTH** Workout

DAY 3

WEEK 6

TODAY'S DATE:	

		1st Circuit			2nd Circuit			3rd Circuit		
		a	b	c	a	b	c	a	b	c
1	Abs/Back	___	/___	/___	___	/___	/___	___	/___	/___

		Warm-Up Set (80%)		Work Set (100%)		Blast Set (80%)	
		Weight	Reps	Weight	Reps	Weight	Reps
2	Bench Press						
3	Lat Pull						
4	Pec Fly						
5	Pulley Row						
6	Lateral Raise						
7	Bicep Curl						
8	Tricep Ext.						
9	Quad Ext.						
10	Hamstring Curl						

Stretched After Workout? ☐

IDEAL ←————————→ **Off Target**

						IDEAL
Water Intake	5	4	3	2	1	+ **Diet**
Fat Intake	5	4	3	2	1	+ **Evaluation**
Protein Intake	5	4	3	2	1	+
Carb Intake	5	4	3	2	1	+
30/40/30%	10	8	6	4	0	=
				TOTAL SCORE		

25–30 = excellent; 19–24 = good; 18 or less = needs work

12ᵀᴴ **CYCLING** Workout

TODAY'S DATE:

Today's Weight:

Average Heart Rate
During Workout:

Total Calories
Burned In
This Workout:

Total Workout
Time:
(Including Warm-Up)

Average Level
Of Intensity:

Stretched After Workout? ☐

**IDEAL
Diet
Evaluation**

IDEAL ←——————→ Off Target

Water Intake	5	4	3	2	1	+
Fat Intake	5	4	3	2	1	+
Protein Intake	5	4	3	2	1	+
Carb Intake	5	4	3	2	1	+
30/40/30%	10	8	6	4	0	=
				TOTAL SCORE		

25–30 = excellent; 19–24 = good; 18 or less = needs work

12ᵀᴴ **RUN/WALK** Workout

TODAY'S DATE:

DAY 5

**WEEK
6**

Average Heart Rate
During Workout:

Total Calories
Burned In
This Workout:
(   ) Miles x 100)

Total Workout
Time:
(Including Warm-Up)

Average Pace

Stretched After Workout? ☐

**IDEAL
Diet
Evaluation**

IDEAL ←——————→ Off Target

Water Intake	5	4	3	2	1	+
Fat Intake	5	4	3	2	1	+
Protein Intake	5	4	3	2	1	+
Carb Intake	5	4	3	2	1	+
30/40/30%	10	8	6	4	0	=
				TOTAL SCORE		

25–30 = excellent; 19–24 = good; 18 or less = needs work

12ᵀᴴ **STRENGTH** Workout

			DAY 6

TODAY'S DATE: _____

		1st Circuit		2nd Circuit		3rd Circuit	
		a b c		a b c		a b c	
1	Abs/Back	__/__/__		__/__/__		__/__/__	

		Warm-Up Set (80%)		Work Set (100%)		Blast Set (80%)	
		Weight	Reps	Weight	Reps	Weight	Reps
2	Bench Press						
3	Lat Pull						
4	Pec Fly						
5	Pulley Row						
6	Lateral Raise						
7	Bicep Curl						
8	Tricep Ext.						
9	Quad Ext.						
10	Hamstring Curl						

Stretched After Workout? ☐

DAY 6

WEEK 6

IDEAL ←————————————→ **Off Target**

Water Intake	5	4	3	2	1	
Fat Intake	5	4	3	2	1	
Protein Intake	5	4	3	2	1	
Carb Intake	5	4	3	2	1	
30/40/30%	10	8	6	4	0	
				TOTAL SCORE		

+ **IDEAL**
+ **Diet**
+ **Evaluation**
+
=

25–30 = excellent; 19–24 = good; 18 or less = needs work

DAY 7 : WEEK 6

DAY OFF!

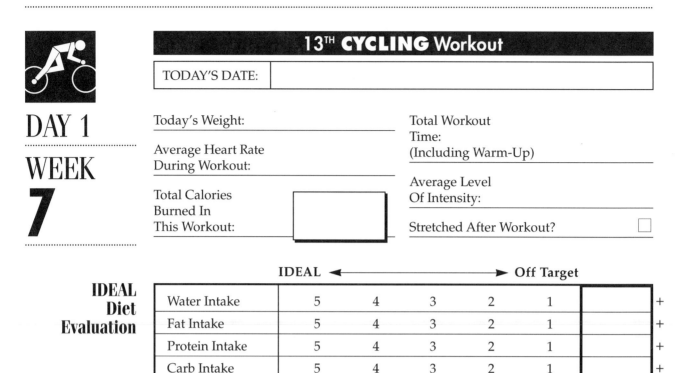

DAY 1
WEEK 7

13ᵀᴴ **CYCLING** Workout

TODAY'S DATE:

Today's Weight:

Average Heart Rate During Workout:

Total Calories Burned In This Workout:

Total Workout Time: (Including Warm-Up)

Average Level Of Intensity:

Stretched After Workout? ☐

IDEAL Diet Evaluation

IDEAL ◄——————► Off Target

Water Intake	5	4	3	2	1	+
Fat Intake	5	4	3	2	1	+
Protein Intake	5	4	3	2	1	+
Carb Intake	5	4	3	2	1	+
30/40/30%	10	8	6	4	0	=
				TOTAL SCORE		

25–30 = excellent; 19–24 = good; 18 or less = needs work

DAY 2
WEEK 7

13ᵀᴴ **RUN/WALK** Workout

TODAY'S DATE:

Average Heart Rate During Workout:

Total Calories Burned In This Workout: (   ) Miles x 100)

Total Workout Time: (Including Warm-Up)

Average Pace

Stretched After Workout? ☐

IDEAL Diet Evaluation

IDEAL ◄——————► Off Target

Water Intake	5	4	3	2	1	+
Fat Intake	5	4	3	2	1	+
Protein Intake	5	4	3	2	1	+
Carb Intake	5	4	3	2	1	+
30/40/30%	10	8	6	4	0	=
				TOTAL SCORE		

25–30 = excellent; 19–24 = good; 18 or less = needs work

148

13ᵀᴴ **STRENGTH** Workout

DAY 3

WEEK

7

TODAY'S DATE:	

		1st Circuit			2nd Circuit			3rd Circuit		
1	Abs/Back	a	b	c	a	b	c	a	b	c
		___	/ ___	/ ___	___	/ ___	/ ___	___	/ ___	/ ___

		Warm-Up Set (80%)		**Work Set (100%)**		**Blast Set (80%)**	
		Weight	Reps	Weight	Reps	Weight	Reps
2	Bench Press						
3	Lat Pull						
4	Pec Fly						
5	Pulley Row						
6	Lateral Raise						
7	Bicep Curl						
8	Tricep Ext.						
9	Quad Ext.						
10	Hamstring Curl						

Stretched After Workout? ☐

	IDEAL ◄————————————► Off Target						
Water Intake	5	4	3	2	1		+
Fat Intake	5	4	3	2	1		+
Protein Intake	5	4	3	2	1		+
Carb Intake	5	4	3	2	1		+
30/40/30%	10	8	6	4	0		=
					TOTAL SCORE		

IDEAL Diet Evaluation

25–30 = excellent; 19–24 = good; 18 or less = needs work

DAY 4

WEEK

7

14ᵀᴴ **CYCLING** Workout

TODAY'S DATE:	

Today's Weight:

Average Heart Rate During Workout:

Total Calories Burned In This Workout:

Total Workout Time: (Including Warm-Up)

Average Level Of Intensity:

Stretched After Workout? ☐

IDEAL Diet Evaluation

IDEAL ◄————————► Off Target

Water Intake	5	4	3	2	1	+
Fat Intake	5	4	3	2	1	+
Protein Intake	5	4	3	2	1	+
Carb Intake	5	4	3	2	1	+
30/40/30%	10	8	6	4	0	=
				TOTAL SCORE		

25–30 = excellent; 19–24 = good; 18 or less = needs work

DAY 5

WEEK

7

14ᵀᴴ **RUN/WALK** Workout

TODAY'S DATE:	

Average Heart Rate During Workout:

Total Calories Burned In This Workout: (   ) Miles x 100)

Total Workout Time: (Including Warm-Up)

Average Pace

Stretched After Workout? ☐

IDEAL Diet Evaluation

IDEAL ◄————————► Off Target

Water Intake	5	4	3	2	1	+
Fat Intake	5	4	3	2	1	+
Protein Intake	5	4	3	2	1	+
Carb Intake	5	4	3	2	1	+
30/40/30%	10	8	6	4	0	=
				TOTAL SCORE		

25–30 = excellent; 19–24 = good; 18 or less = needs work

150

14ᵀᴴ **STRENGTH** Workout

DAY 6

WEEK 7

TODAY'S DATE:	

		1st Circuit			2nd Circuit			3rd Circuit		
1	Abs/Back	a ___	b ___	c ___	a ___	b ___	c ___	a ___	b ___	c ___

		Warm-Up Set (80%)		Work Set (100%)		Blast Set (80%)	
		Weight	Reps	Weight	Reps	Weight	Reps
2	Bench Press						
3	Lat Pull						
4	Pec Fly						
5	Pulley Row						
6	Lateral Raise						
7	Bicep Curl						
8	Tricep Ext.						
9	Quad Ext.						
10	Hamstring Curl						

Stretched After Workout? ☐

IDEAL ⟷ **Off Target**

Water Intake	5	4	3	2	1		+
Fat Intake	5	4	3	2	1		+
Protein Intake	5	4	3	2	1		+
Carb Intake	5	4	3	2	1		+
30/40/30%	10	8	6	4	0		=
				TOTAL SCORE			

IDEAL Diet Evaluation

25–30 = excellent; 19–24 = good; 18 or less = needs work

DAY 7: WEEK 7

DAY OFF!

15ᵀᴴ **CYCLING** Workout

DAY 1

WEEK 8

TODAY'S DATE:

Today's Weight:

Average Heart Rate During Workout:

Total Calories Burned In This Workout:

Total Workout Time: (Including Warm-Up)

Average Level Of Intensity:

Stretched After Workout? ☐

IDEAL Diet Evaluation

	IDEAL ←——————→ Off Target						
Water Intake	5	4	3	2	1		+
Fat Intake	5	4	3	2	1		+
Protein Intake	5	4	3	2	1		+
Carb Intake	5	4	3	2	1		+
30/40/30%	10	8	6	4	0		=
					TOTAL SCORE		

25–30 = excellent; 19–24 = good; 18 or less = needs work

15ᵀᴴ **RUN/WALK** Workout

DAY 2

WEEK 8

TODAY'S DATE:

Average Heart Rate During Workout:

Total Calories Burned In This Workout: (   ) Miles x 100)

Total Workout Time: (Including Warm-Up)

Average Pace

Stretched After Workout? ☐

IDEAL Diet Evaluation

	IDEAL ←——————→ Off Target						
Water Intake	5	4	3	2	1		+
Fat Intake	5	4	3	2	1		+
Protein Intake	5	4	3	2	1		+
Carb Intake	5	4	3	2	1		+
30/40/30%	10	8	6	4	0		=
					TOTAL SCORE		

25–30 = excellent; 19–24 = good; 18 or less = needs work

15ᵀᴴ **STRENGTH** Workout

DAY 3

WEEK

8

TODAY'S DATE:	

		1st Circuit			2nd Circuit			3rd Circuit		
		a	b	c	a	b	c	a	b	c
1	Abs/Back	__/__/__			__/__/__			__/__/__		

		Warm-Up Set (80%)		Work Set (100%)		Blast Set (80%)	
		Weight	Reps	Weight	Reps	Weight	Reps
2	Bench Press						
3	Lat Pull						
4	Pec Fly						
5	Pulley Row						
6	Lateral Raise						
7	Bicep Curl						
8	Tricep Ext.						
9	Quad Ext.						
10	Hamstring Curl						

Stretched After Workout? ☐

IDEAL ←—————→ Off Target

Water Intake	5	4	3	2	1		+
Fat Intake	5	4	3	2	1		+
Protein Intake	5	4	3	2	1		+
Carb Intake	5	4	3	2	1		+
30/40/30%	10	8	6	4	0		=
				TOTAL SCORE		

IDEAL Diet Evaluation

25–30 = excellent; 19–24 = good; 18 or less = needs work

DAY 4
WEEK
8

16ᵀᴴ **CYCLING** Workout

TODAY'S DATE:

Today's Weight:

Average Heart Rate
During Workout:

Total Calories
Burned In
This Workout:

Total Workout
Time:
(Including Warm-Up)

Average Level
Of Intensity:

Stretched After Workout? ☐

IDEAL Diet Evaluation

IDEAL ←————————→ Off Target

Water Intake	5	4	3	2	1	+
Fat Intake	5	4	3	2	1	+
Protein Intake	5	4	3	2	1	+
Carb Intake	5	4	3	2	1	+
30/40/30%	10	8	6	4	0	=
				TOTAL SCORE		

25–30 = excellent; 19–24 = good; 18 or less = needs work

DAY 5
WEEK
8

16ᵀᴴ **RUN/WALK** Workout

TODAY'S DATE:

Average Heart Rate
During Workout:

Total Calories
Burned In
This Workout:
(   ) Miles x 100)

Total Workout
Time:
(Including Warm-Up)

Average Pace

Stretched After Workout? ☐

IDEAL Diet Evaluation

IDEAL ←————————→ Off Target

Water Intake	5	4	3	2	1	+
Fat Intake	5	4	3	2	1	+
Protein Intake	5	4	3	2	1	+
Carb Intake	5	4	3	2	1	+
30/40/30%	10	8	6	4	0	=
				TOTAL SCORE		

25–30 = excellent; 19–24 = good; 18 or less = needs work

16ᵀᴴ **STRENGTH** Workout

DAY 6

WEEK 8

TODAY'S DATE:	

		1st Circuit			2nd Circuit			3rd Circuit		
1	Abs/Back	a	b	c	a	b	c	a	b	c
		__/__/__			__/__/__			__/__/__		

		Warm-Up Set (80%)		Work Set (100%)		Blast Set (80%)	
		Weight	Reps	Weight	Reps	Weight	Reps
2	Bench Press						
3	Lat Pull						
4	Pec Fly						
5	Pulley Row						
6	Lateral Raise						
7	Bicep Curl						
8	Tricep Ext.						
9	Quad Ext.						
10	Hamstring Curl						

Stretched After Workout? ☐

IDEAL ⟵──────────⟶ **Off Target**

Water Intake	5	4	3	2	1	+
Fat Intake	5	4	3	2	1	+
Protein Intake	5	4	3	2	1	+
Carb Intake	5	4	3	2	1	+
30/40/30%	10	8	6	4	0	=
				TOTAL SCORE		

IDEAL Diet Evaluation

25–30 = excellent; 19–24 = good; 18 or less = needs work

DAY 7 : WEEK 8

DAY OFF!

DAY 1
WEEK
9

17ᵀᴴ **CYCLING** Workout

TODAY'S DATE:

Today's Weight:

Average Heart Rate
During Workout:

Total Calories
Burned In
This Workout:

Total Workout
Time:
(Including Warm-Up)

Average Level
Of Intensity:

Stretched After Workout? ☐

IDEAL Diet Evaluation

IDEAL ◄─────────► Off Target

Water Intake	5	4	3	2	1	+
Fat Intake	5	4	3	2	1	+
Protein Intake	5	4	3	2	1	+
Carb Intake	5	4	3	2	1	+
30/40/30%	10	8	6	4	0	=
					TOTAL SCORE	

25–30 = excellent; 19–24 = good; 18 or less = needs work

DAY 2
WEEK
9

17ᵀᴴ **RUN/WALK** Workout

TODAY'S DATE:

Average Heart Rate
During Workout:

Total Calories
Burned In
This Workout:
(   ) Miles x 100)

Total Workout
Time:
(Including Warm-Up)

Average Pace

Stretched After Workout? ☐

IDEAL Diet Evaluation

IDEAL ◄─────────► Off Target

Water Intake	5	4	3	2	1	+
Fat Intake	5	4	3	2	1	+
Protein Intake	5	4	3	2	1	+
Carb Intake	5	4	3	2	1	+
30/40/30%	10	8	6	4	0	=
					TOTAL SCORE	

25–30 = excellent; 19–24 = good; 18 or less = needs work

17ᵀᴴ **STRENGTH** Workout

	1st Circuit			2nd Circuit			3rd Circuit		
	a	b	c	a	b	c	a	b	c
1 Abs/Back	___ / ___ / ___			___ / ___ / ___			___ / ___ / ___		

TODAY'S DATE: _____

DAY 3

WEEK 9

	Warm-Up Set (80%)		Work Set (100%)		Blast Set (80%)	
	Weight	Reps	Weight	Reps	Weight	Reps
2 Bench Press						
3 Lat Pull						
4 Pec Fly						
5 Pulley Row						
6 Lateral Raise						
7 Bicep Curl						
8 Tricep Ext.						
9 Quad Ext.						
10 Hamstring Curl						

Stretched After Workout? ☐

	IDEAL ←⎯⎯⎯⎯⎯⎯→ Off Target						
Water Intake	5	4	3	2	1		+ **IDEAL**
Fat Intake	5	4	3	2	1		+ **Diet**
Protein Intake	5	4	3	2	1		+ **Evaluation**
Carb Intake	5	4	3	2	1		+
30/40/30%	10	8	6	4	0		=
				TOTAL SCORE			

25–30 = excellent; 19–24 = good; 18 or less = needs work

18ᵀᴴ **CYCLING** Workout

TODAY'S DATE:

Today's Weight:

Average Heart Rate
During Workout:

Total Calories
Burned In
This Workout:

Total Workout
Time:
(Including Warm-Up)

Average Level
Of Intensity:

Stretched After Workout? ☐

DAY 4

WEEK 9

IDEAL Diet Evaluation

	IDEAL ⟵			⟶ Off Target			
Water Intake	5	4	3	2	1		+
Fat Intake	5	4	3	2	1		+
Protein Intake	5	4	3	2	1		+
Carb Intake	5	4	3	2	1		+
30/40/30%	10	8	6	4	0		=
					TOTAL SCORE		

25–30 = excellent; 19–24 = good; 18 or less = needs work

18ᵀᴴ **RUN/WALK** Workout

TODAY'S DATE:

Average Heart Rate
During Workout:

Total Calories
Burned In
This Workout:
(   ) Miles x 100)

Total Workout
Time:
(Including Warm-Up)

Average Pace

Stretched After Workout? ☐

DAY 5

WEEK 9

IDEAL Diet Evaluation

	IDEAL ⟵			⟶ Off Target			
Water Intake	5	4	3	2	1		+
Fat Intake	5	4	3	2	1		+
Protein Intake	5	4	3	2	1		+
Carb Intake	5	4	3	2	1		+
30/40/30%	10	8	6	4	0		=
					TOTAL SCORE		

25–30 = excellent; 19–24 = good; 18 or less = needs work

18ᵀᴴ **STRENGTH** Workout

TODAY'S DATE: _____

DAY 6

WEEK

9

		1st Circuit			2nd Circuit			3rd Circuit		
1	Abs/Back	a ___	b ___	c ___	a ___	b ___	c ___	a ___	b ___	c ___

		Warm-Up Set (80%)		**Work Set (100%)**		**Blast Set (80%)**	
		Weight	Reps	Weight	Reps	Weight	Reps
2	Bench Press						
3	Lat Pull						
4	Pec Fly						
5	Pulley Row						
6	Lateral Raise						
7	Bicep Curl						
8	Tricep Ext.						
9	Quad Ext.						
10	Hamstring Curl						

Stretched After Workout? ☐

	IDEAL ←			→ Off Target		
Water Intake	5	4	3	2	1	+
Fat Intake	5	4	3	2	1	+
Protein Intake	5	4	3	2	1	+
Carb Intake	5	4	3	2	1	+
30/40/30%	10	8	6	4	0	=
				TOTAL SCORE		

IDEAL Diet Evaluation

25–30 = excellent; 19–24 = good; 18 or less = needs work

DAY 7: WEEK 9

DAY OFF

DAY 1
WEEK
10

19TH **CYCLING** Workout

TODAY'S DATE:

Today's Weight:

Average Heart Rate
During Workout:

Total Calories
Burned In
This Workout:

Total Workout
Time:
(Including Warm-Up)

Average Level
Of Intensity:

Stretched After Workout? ☐

IDEAL Diet Evaluation

	IDEAL ←			→ Off Target			
Water Intake	5	4	3	2	1		+
Fat Intake	5	4	3	2	1		+
Protein Intake	5	4	3	2	1		+
Carb Intake	5	4	3	2	1		+
30/40/30%	10	8	6	4	0		=
					TOTAL SCORE		

25–30 = excellent; 19–24 = good; 18 or less = needs work

DAY 2
WEEK
10

19TH **RUN/WALK** Workout

TODAY'S DATE:

Average Heart Rate
During Workout:

Total Calories
Burned In
This Workout:
(   ) Miles x 100)

Total Workout
Time:
(Including Warm-Up)

Average Pace

Stretched After Workout? ☐

IDEAL Diet Evaluation

	IDEAL ←			→ Off Target			
Water Intake	5	4	3	2	1		+
Fat Intake	5	4	3	2	1		+
Protein Intake	5	4	3	2	1		+
Carb Intake	5	4	3	2	1		+
30/40/30%	10	8	6	4	0		=
					TOTAL SCORE		

25–30 = excellent; 19–24 = good; 18 or less = needs work

19ᵀᴴ **STRENGTH** Workout

DAY 3

WEEK 10

TODAY'S DATE:	

		1st Circuit			2nd Circuit			3rd Circuit		
1	Abs/Back	a	b	c	a	b	c	a	b	c
		__/__ /__			__/__ /__			__/__ /__		

		Warm-Up Set (80%)		**Work Set (100%)**		**Blast Set (80%)**	
		Weight	Reps	Weight	Reps	Weight	Reps
2	Bench Press						
3	Lat Pull						
4	Pec Fly						
5	Pulley Row						
6	Lateral Raise						
7	Bicep Curl						
8	Tricep Ext.						
9	Quad Ext.						
10	Hamstring Curl						

Stretched After Workout? ☐

IDEAL ←⎯⎯⎯⎯⎯⎯→ **Off Target**

	IDEAL				Off Target	
Water Intake	5	4	3	2	1	
Fat Intake	5	4	3	2	1	
Protein Intake	5	4	3	2	1	
Carb Intake	5	4	3	2	1	
30/40/30%	10	8	6	4	0	
				TOTAL SCORE		

IDEAL Diet Evaluation

+
+
+
+
=

25–30 = excellent; 19–24 = good; 18 or less = needs work

161

DAY 4

WEEK
10

20ᵀᴴ CYCLING Workout

TODAY'S DATE:

Today's Weight:

Average Heart Rate
During Workout:

Total Calories
Burned In
This Workout:

Total Workout
Time:
(Including Warm-Up)

Average Level
Of Intensity:

Stretched After Workout? ☐

IDEAL
Diet
Evaluation

	IDEAL ◄――――――► Off Target						
Water Intake	5	4	3	2	1		+
Fat Intake	5	4	3	2	1		+
Protein Intake	5	4	3	2	1		+
Carb Intake	5	4	3	2	1		+
30/40/30%	10	8	6	4	0		=
				TOTAL SCORE			

25–30 = excellent; 19–24 = good; 18 or less = needs work

DAY 5

WEEK
10

20ᵀᴴ RUN/WALK Workout

TODAY'S DATE:

Average Heart Rate
During Workout:

Total Calories
Burned In
This Workout:
(   ) Miles x 100)

Total Workout
Time:
(Including Warm-Up)

Average Pace

Stretched After Workout? ☐

IDEAL
Diet
Evaluation

	IDEAL ◄――――――► Off Target						
Water Intake	5	4	3	2	1		+
Fat Intake	5	4	3	2	1		+
Protein Intake	5	4	3	2	1		+
Carb Intake	5	4	3	2	1		+
30/40/30%	10	8	6	4	0		=
				TOTAL SCORE			

25–30 = excellent; 19–24 = good; 18 or less = needs work

20TH **STRENGTH** Workout

TODAY'S DATE:	

DAY 6

WEEK

10

		1st Circuit			2nd Circuit			3rd Circuit		
		a	b	c	a	b	c	a	b	c
1	Abs/Back	___/___/___			___/___/___			___/___/___		

		Warm-Up Set (80%)		Work Set (100%)		Blast Set (80%)	
		Weight	Reps	Weight	Reps	Weight	Reps
2	Bench Press						
3	Lat Pull						
4	Pec Fly						
5	Pulley Row						
6	Lateral Raise						
7	Bicep Curl						
8	Tricep Ext.						
9	Quad Ext.						
10	Hamstring Curl						

Stretched After Workout? ☐

	IDEAL ⬅			➡ Off Target			
Water Intake	5	4	3	2	1		+
Fat Intake	5	4	3	2	1		+
Protein Intake	5	4	3	2	1		+
Carb Intake	5	4	3	2	1		+
30/40/30%	10	8	6	4	0		=
				TOTAL SCORE			

IDEAL Diet Evaluation

25–30 = excellent; 19–24 = good; 18 or less = needs work

DAY 7 : WEEK 10

DAY OFF!

DAY 1
WEEK
11

21ST **CYCLING** Workout

TODAY'S DATE:

Today's Weight:

Average Heart Rate
During Workout:

Total Calories
Burned In
This Workout:

Total Workout
Time:
(Including Warm-Up)

Average Level
Of Intensity:

Stretched After Workout? ☐

**IDEAL
Diet
Evaluation**

	IDEAL ←			→ Off	Target		
Water Intake	5	4	3	2	1		+
Fat Intake	5	4	3	2	1		+
Protein Intake	5	4	3	2	1		+
Carb Intake	5	4	3	2	1		+
30/40/30%	10	8	6	4	0		=
					TOTAL SCORE		

25–30 = excellent; 19–24 = good; 18 or less = needs work

DAY 2
WEEK
11

21ST **RUN/WALK** Workout

TODAY'S DATE:

Average Heart Rate
During Workout:

Total Calories
Burned In
This Workout:
(   ) Miles x 100)

Total Workout
Time:
(Including Warm-Up)

Average Pace

Stretched After Workout? ☐

**IDEAL
Diet
Evaluation**

	IDEAL ←			→ Off	Target		
Water Intake	5	4	3	2	1		+
Fat Intake	5	4	3	2	1		+
Protein Intake	5	4	3	2	1		+
Carb Intake	5	4	3	2	1		+
30/40/30%	10	8	6	4	0		=
					TOTAL SCORE		

25–30 = excellent; 19–24 = good; 18 or less = needs work

21ST **STRENGTH** Workout

TODAY'S DATE:

DAY 3

WEEK

11

		1st Circuit			2nd Circuit			3rd Circuit		
		a	b	c	a	b	c	a	b	c
1	Abs/Back	__/__/__			__/__/__			__/__/__		

		Warm-Up Set (80%)		Work Set (100%)		Blast Set (80%)	
		Weight	Reps	Weight	Reps	Weight	Reps
2	Bench Press						
3	Lat Pull						
4	Pec Fly						
5	Pulley Row						
6	Lateral Raise						
7	Bicep Curl						
8	Tricep Ext.						
9	Quad Ext.						
10	Hamstring Curl						

Stretched After Workout? ☐

	IDEAL ←——————→ Off Target						
Water Intake	5	4	3	2	1		+
Fat Intake	5	4	3	2	1		+
Protein Intake	5	4	3	2	1		+
Carb Intake	5	4	3	2	1		+
30/40/30%	10	8	6	4	0		=
				TOTAL SCORE			

IDEAL Diet Evaluation

25–30 = excellent; 19–24 = good; 18 or less = needs work

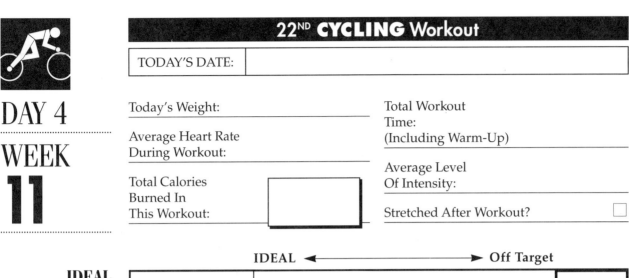

DAY 4
WEEK 11

22ND CYCLING Workout

TODAY'S DATE:

Today's Weight:

Average Heart Rate
During Workout:

Total Calories
Burned In
This Workout:

Total Workout
Time:
(Including Warm-Up)

Average Level
Of Intensity:

Stretched After Workout? ☐

IDEAL Diet Evaluation

	IDEAL ←			→ Off Target			
Water Intake	5	4	3	2	1		+
Fat Intake	5	4	3	2	1		+
Protein Intake	5	4	3	2	1		+
Carb Intake	5	4	3	2	1		+
30/40/30%	10	8	6	4	0		=
					TOTAL SCORE		

25–30 = excellent; 19–24 = good; 18 or less = needs work

DAY 5
WEEK 11

22ND RUN/WALK Workout

TODAY'S DATE:

Average Heart Rate
During Workout:

Total Calories
Burned In
This Workout:
(   ) Miles x 100)

Total Workout
Time:
(Including Warm-Up)

Average Pace

Stretched After Workout? ☐

IDEAL Diet Evaluation

	IDEAL ←			→ Off Target			
Water Intake	5	4	3	2	1		+
Fat Intake	5	4	3	2	1		+
Protein Intake	5	4	3	2	1		+
Carb Intake	5	4	3	2	1		+
30/40/30%	10	8	6	4	0		=
					TOTAL SCORE		

25–30 = excellent; 19–24 = good; 18 or less = needs work

22ND **STRENGTH** Workout

DAY 6

WEEK 11

TODAY'S DATE:	

		1st Circuit			2nd Circuit			3rd Circuit		
1	Abs/Back	a	b	c	a	b	c	a	b	c
		___/___/___			___/___/___			___/___/___		

		Warm-Up Set (80%)		**Work Set (100%)**		**Blast Set (80%)**	
		Weight	Reps	Weight	Reps	Weight	Reps
2	Bench Press						
3	Lat Pull						
4	Pec Fly						
5	Pulley Row						
6	Lateral Raise						
7	Bicep Curl						
8	Tricep Ext.						
9	Quad Ext.						
10	Hamstring Curl						

Stretched After Workout? ☐

IDEAL ←————————→ **Off Target**

Water Intake	5	4	3	2	1		+
Fat Intake	5	4	3	2	1		+
Protein Intake	5	4	3	2	1		+
Carb Intake	5	4	3	2	1		+
30/40/30%	10	8	6	4	0		=
				TOTAL SCORE			

IDEAL Diet Evaluation

25–30 = excellent; 19–24 = good; 18 or less = needs work

DAY 7: WEEK 11

DAY OFF!

DAY 1
WEEK
12

23ᴿᴰ **CYCLING** Workout

TODAY'S DATE:

Today's Weight:

Average Heart Rate
During Workout:

Total Calories
Burned In
This Workout:

Total Workout
Time:
(Including Warm-Up)

Average Level
Of Intensity:

Stretched After Workout? ☐

**IDEAL
Diet
Evaluation**

	IDEAL ←———————→ Off Target						
Water Intake	5	4	3	2	1		+
Fat Intake	5	4	3	2	1		+
Protein Intake	5	4	3	2	1		+
Carb Intake	5	4	3	2	1		+
30/40/30%	10	8	6	4	0		=
					TOTAL SCORE		

25–30 = excellent; 19–24 = good; 18 or less = needs work

DAY 2
WEEK
12

23ᴿᴰ **RUN/WALK** Workout

TODAY'S DATE:

Average Heart Rate
During Workout:

Total Calories
Burned In
This Workout:
(   ) Miles x 100)

Total Workout
Time:
(Including Warm-Up)

Average Pace

Stretched After Workout? ☐

**IDEAL
Diet
Evaluation**

	IDEAL ←———————→ Off Target						
Water Intake	5	4	3	2	1		+
Fat Intake	5	4	3	2	1		+
Protein Intake	5	4	3	2	1		+
Carb Intake	5	4	3	2	1		+
30/40/30%	10	8	6	4	0		=
					TOTAL SCORE		

25–30 = excellent; 19–24 = good; 18 or less = needs work

23RD STRENGTH Workout

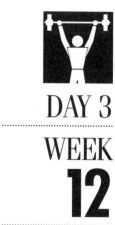

DAY 3

WEEK

12

TODAY'S DATE:	

		1st Circuit			2nd Circuit			3rd Circuit		
1	**Abs/Back**	a	b	c	a	b	c	a	b	c
		___/___/___			___/___/___			___/___/___		

		Warm-Up Set (80%)		Work Set (100%)		Blast Set (80%)	
		Weight	Reps	Weight	Reps	Weight	Reps
2	Bench Press						
3	Lat Pull						
4	Pec Fly						
5	Pulley Row						
6	Lateral Raise						
7	Bicep Curl						
8	Tricep Ext.						
9	Quad Ext.						
10	Hamstring Curl						

Stretched After Workout? ☐

IDEAL ←——————————→ **Off Target**

Water Intake	5	4	3	2	1		+ **IDEAL**
Fat Intake	5	4	3	2	1		+ **Diet**
Protein Intake	5	4	3	2	1		+ **Evaluation**
Carb Intake	5	4	3	2	1		+
30/40/30%	10	8	6	4	0		=
				TOTAL SCORE			

25–30 = excellent; 19–24 = good; 18 or less = needs work

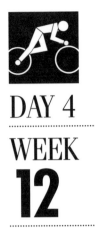

DAY 4

WEEK 12

24TH **CYCLING** Workout

TODAY'S DATE:

Today's Weight:

Average Heart Rate
During Workout:

Total Calories
Burned In
This Workout:

Total Workout
Time:
(Including Warm-Up)

Average Level
Of Intensity:

Stretched After Workout? ☐

IDEAL Diet Evaluation

	IDEAL ←			→ Off Target			
Water Intake	5	4	3	2	1		+
Fat Intake	5	4	3	2	1		+
Protein Intake	5	4	3	2	1		+
Carb Intake	5	4	3	2	1		+
30/40/30%	10	8	6	4	0		=
					TOTAL SCORE		

25–30 = excellent; 19–24 = good; 18 or less = needs work

DAY 5

WEEK 12

24TH **RUN/WALK** Workout

TODAY'S DATE:

Average Heart Rate
During Workout:

Total Calories
Burned In
This Workout:
(   ) Miles x 100)

Total Workout
Time:
(Including Warm-Up)

Average Pace

Stretched After Workout? ☐

IDEAL Diet Evaluation

	IDEAL ←			→ Off Target			
Water Intake	5	4	3	2	1		+
Fat Intake	5	4	3	2	1		+
Protein Intake	5	4	3	2	1		+
Carb Intake	5	4	3	2	1		+
30/40/30%	10	8	6	4	0		=
					TOTAL SCORE		

25–30 = excellent; 19–24 = good; 18 or less = needs work

24ᵀᴴ **STRENGTH** Workout

DAY 6

WEEK 12

	TODAY'S DATE:	

		1st Circuit			2nd Circuit			3rd Circuit		
1	Abs/Back	a	b	c	a	b	c	a	b	c
		___/___/___			___/___/___			___/___/___		
		Warm-Up Set (80%)		**Work Set (100%)**		**Blast Set (80%)**	
		Weight	Reps	Weight	Reps	Weight	Reps
2	Bench Press						
3	Lat Pull						
4	Pec Fly						
5	Pulley Row						
6	Lateral Raise						
7	Bicep Curl						
8	Tricep Ext.						
9	Quad Ext.						
10	Hamstring Curl						

Stretched After Workout? ☐

	IDEAL ←⟶ Off Target						
Water Intake	5	4	3	2	1		+
Fat Intake	5	4	3	2	1		+
Protein Intake	5	4	3	2	1		+
Carb Intake	5	4	3	2	1		+
30/40/30%	10	8	6	4	0		=
				TOTAL SCORE			

IDEAL Diet Evaluation

25–30 = excellent; 19–24 = good; 18 or less = needs work

DAY 7 : WEEK 12

DAY OFF

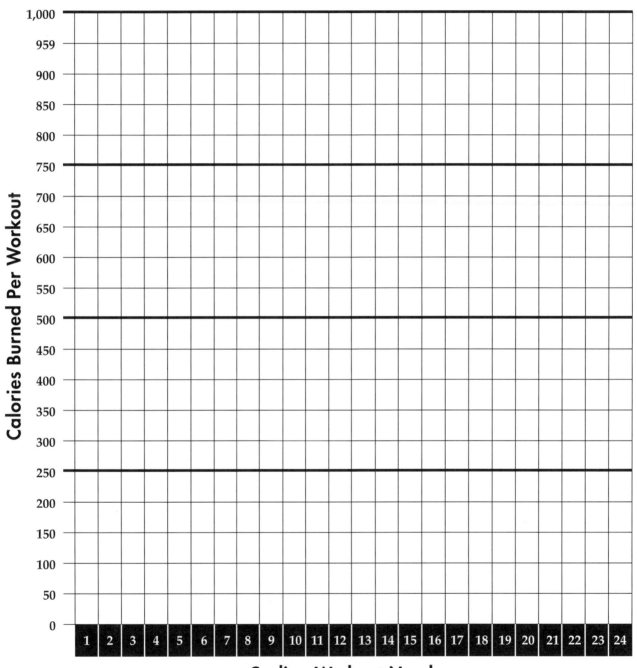

12-Week **CYCLING** Progress Chart

Calories Burned Per Workout

1,000
959
900
850
800
750
700
650
600
550
500
450
400
350
300
250
200
150
100
50
0

| 1 | 2 | 3 | 4 | 5 | 6 | 7 | 8 | 9 | 10 | 11 | 12 | 13 | 14 | 15 | 16 | 17 | 18 | 19 | 20 | 21 | 22 | 23 | 24 |

Cycling Workout Number

12-Week RUNNING/WALKING Progress Chart

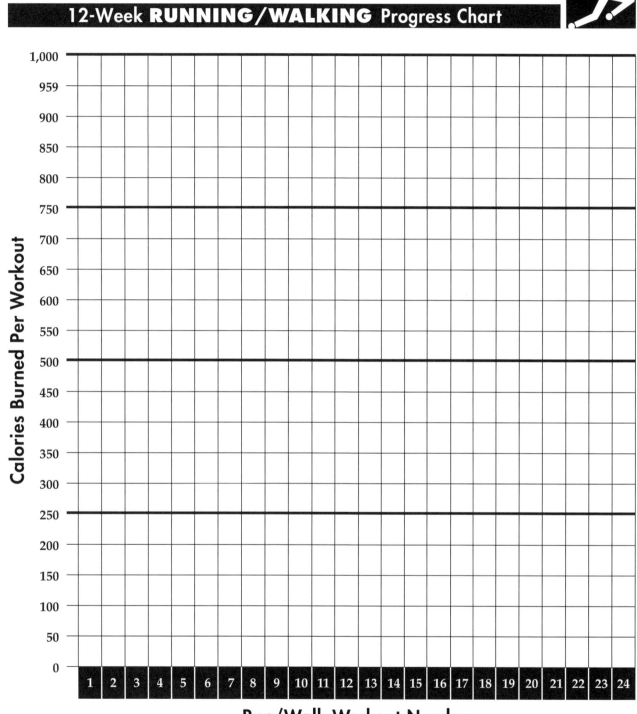

Calories Burned Per Workout

1,000
959
900
850
800
750
700
650
600
550
500
450
400
350
300
250
200
150
100
50
0

| 1 | 2 | 3 | 4 | 5 | 6 | 7 | 8 | 9 | 10 | 11 | 12 | 13 | 14 | 15 | 16 | 17 | 18 | 19 | 20 | 21 | 22 | 23 | 24 |

Run/Walk Workout Number

12-Week INCREASE IN STRENGTH

	A	B	C	Percent Gain in Strength			
	Ten-rep max. Workout 24	Ten-rep max. Workout 3	Difference A-B	(C)	÷	(B) (x 100) =	%
Bench Press				(C)		(B)	
				_____ ÷ _____ (x 100)=_____ %			
Lat Pull				(C)		(B)	
				_____ ÷ _____ (x 100)=_____ %			
Pec Fly				(C)		(B)	
				_____ ÷ _____ (x 100)=_____ %			
Pulley Row				(C)		(B)	
				_____ ÷ _____ (x 100)=_____ %			
Lateral Raise				(C)		(B)	
				_____ ÷ _____ (x 100)=_____ %			
Bicep Curl				(C)		(B)	
				_____ ÷ _____ (x 100)=_____ %			
Tricep Extension				(C)		(B)	
				_____ ÷ _____ (x 100)=_____ %			
Quad Extension				(C)		(B)	
				_____ ÷ _____ (x 100)=_____ %			
Hamstring Curl				(C)		(B)	
				_____ ÷ _____ (x 100)=_____ %			

12-Week **IMPROVEMENT SUMMARY**

Use the following formulas to evaluate exactly how much you have accomplished over the 12 weeks.

FAT LOSS

1.   Starting Body Fat   Ending Body Fat   Fat Lost

_____ pounds   −   _____ pounds   =   _____ pounds

2.   Fat Lost   Starting Body Fat   Percent Body Fat Lost

_____ pounds   ÷   _____ pounds   x 100 =   _____ %

INCREASE IN AEROBIC CAPACITY

1.   Total Calories Burned   Total Calories Burned   Increase in Calories
         in Last 60-Minute   in First 60-Minute   Burned for
         Cycling Workout   Cycling Workout   60 Minutes

_____   −   _____   =   _____

2.   Increase in   Calories Burned   Percent Increase
         Calories   In First Workout   in Aerobic Capacity

_____   ÷   _____   x 100 =   _____

INCREASE IN STRENGTH (*on each piece of equipment*):

1.   Ten-Rep Max   Ten-Rep Max   Increase In
         In Final Workout   In Third Workout   Ten-Rep Max

_____ pounds   −   _____ pounds   =   _____ pounds

2.   Increase In   Ten-Rep Max   Percent Increase
         Ten-Rep Max   In Third Workout   in Strength

_____ pounds   ÷   _____ pounds   x 100 =   _____ %

BODY FAT Interpretation Chart

(as a percentage of total body weight)

MALES (mm)

Age In Years	2-3	4-5	6-7	8-9	10-11	12-13	14-15	16-17	18-19	20-21	22-23	24-25	26-27	28-29	30-31	32-33	34-35
Up to 20	2.0	3.9	6.2	8.5	10.5	12.5	14.3	16.0	17.5	18.9	20.2	21.3	22.3	23.1	23.8	24.3	24.9
21 – 25	2.5	4.9	7.3	9.5	11.6	13.6	15.4	17.0	18.6	20.0	21.2	22.3	23.3	24.2	24.9	25.4	25.8
26 – 30	3.5	6.0	8.4	10.6	12.7	14.6	16.4	18.1	19.6	21.0	22.3	23.4	24.4	25.2	25.9	26.5	26.9
31 – 35	4.5	7.1	9.4	11.7	13.7	15.7	17.5	19.2	20.7	22.1	23.4	24.5	25.5	26.3	27.0	27.5	28.0
36 – 40	5.6	8.1	10.5	12.7	14.8	16.8	18.6	20.2	21.8	23.2	24.4	25.6	26.5	27.4	28.1	28.6	29.0
41 – 45	6.7	9.2	11.5	13.8	15.9	17.8	19.6	21.3	22.8	24.7	25.5	26.6	27.6	28.4	29.1	29.7	30.1
46 – 50	7.7	10.2	12.6	14.8	16.9	18.9	20.7	22.4	23.9	25.3	26.6	27.7	28.7	29.5	30.2	30.7	31.2
51 – 55	8.8	11.3	13.7	15.9	18.0	20.0	21.8	23.4	25.0	26.4	27.6	28.7	29.7	30.6	31.2	31.8	32.2
56 – up	9.9	12.4	14.7	17.0	19.1	21.0	22.8	24.5	26.0	27.4	28.7	29.8	30.8	31.6	32.3	32.9	33.3

FEMALES (mm)

Age In Years	2-3	4-5	6-7	8-9	10-11	12-13	14-15	16-17	18-19	20-21	22-23	24-25	26-27	28-29	30-31	32-33	34-35
Up to 20	11.3	13.5	15.7	17.7	19.7	21.5	23.2	24.8	26.3	27.7	29.0	30.2	31.3	32.3	33.1	33.9	34.6
21 – 25	11.9	14.2	16.3	18.4	20.3	22.1	23.8	25.5	27.0	28.4	29.6	30.8	31.9	32.9	33.8	34.5	35.2
26 – 30	12.5	14.8	16.9	19.0	20.9	22.7	24.5	26.1	27.6	29.0	30.3	31.5	32.5	33.5	34.4	35.2	35.8
31 – 35	13.2	15.4	17.6	19.6	21.5	23.4	25.1	26.7	28.2	29.6	30.9	32.1	33.2	34.1	35.0	35.8	36.4
36 – 40	13.8	16.0	18.2	20.2	22.2	24.0	25.7	27.3	28.8	30.2	31.5	32.7	33.8	34.8	35.6	36.4	37.0
41 – 45	14.4	16.7	18.8	20.8	22.8	24.6	26.3	27.9	29.4	30.8	32.1	33.3	34.4	35.4	36.3	37.0	37.7
46 – 50	15.0	17.3	19.4	21.5	23.4	25.2	26.9	28.6	30.1	31.5	32.8	34.0	35.0	36.0	36.9	37.6	38.3
51 – 55	15.6	17.9	20.0	22.1	24.0	25.9	27.6	29.2	30.7	32.1	33.4	34.6	35.6	36.6	37.5	38.3	38.9
56 – up	16.3	18.5	20.7	22.7	24.6	26.5	28.2	29.8	31.3	32.7	34.0	35.2	36.3	37.2	38.1	38.9	39.5

☐ Lean ▨ Ideal ▨ Average ▨ Overfat

© Accu-Measure 1991

Please call 310-471-7360 for information regarding our unique protein powder's anti-oxident supplements or our new, exclusive line of low-fat California fitnuts.